PEDIATRIC PHYSICAL THERAPY STRENGTHENING EXERCISES FOR THE ANKLES

PEDIATRIC PHYSICAL THERAPY STRENGTHENING EXERCISES FOR THE ANKLES

Treatment Suggestions
by
Muscle Action

Amy E. Sturkey, PT

For information contact:
Amy E. Sturkey, PT
amysturkey@gmail.com
www.igotchaapps.com

Book and Cover design by Guy Bryant

ISBN-13:978-0-9981567-8-1
First Edition: January 20201

DEDICATION

This book is dedicated to all PT students who asked for treatment ideas and every mother who wanted help for her child.

CONTENTS

I. PLANTARFLEXION

THE ANKLE PLANTARFLEXORS MOVE THE top of the foot away from the leg. Activating your plantarflexors makes you stand on your tiptoes or point your toes. Weakness in the plantarflexors makes it harder to jump, run, or walk, especially on uneven surfaces. As pediatric physical therapists, we often deal with stiffness or spasticity in the plantarflexor group associated with cerebral palsy or toe walking. A spastic or stiff muscle has poor voluntary control of the strength, power, or coordination of the movement. This chapter includes a wide variety of exercises to improve ankle plantarflexor strength and control.

* * *

1. BOUNCING SITTING ON A BALL

Long before a child can jump, she can bounce sitting on a ball. I try to use a ball that is about the height of the back of the child's knees. Sometimes the right height is hard to find. If the ball is too short, I can put a bench or a mat under the ball. If the ball is too tall, I put a bench or mat under the feet to get 90 degrees knee flexion and 90 degrees hip flexion. Watch out for substitutions. Lots of kids will substitute trunk movement instead of ankle work.

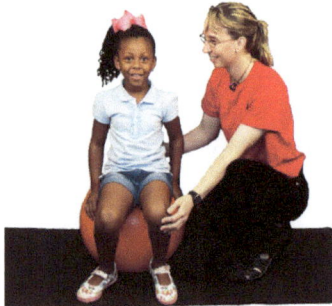

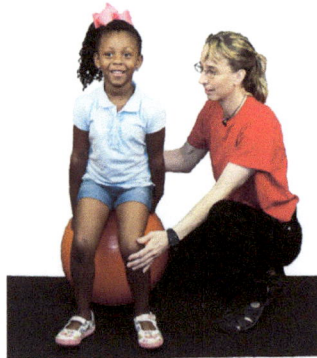

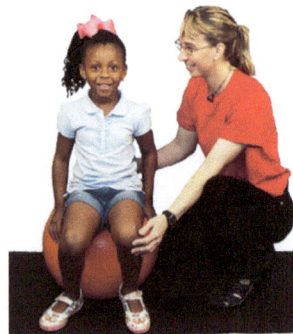

2. SIT TO STAND

To answer your question, yes. Yes, I do think this is a plantarflexion exercise. If you get movement at a joint, you likely get muscle activation. The more movement at the joint, the more likely there is muscle activation. If I am trying to get plantarflexion, I scoot the client forward on the seat. I place the feet a little further back so there is more than 90 degrees knee flexion. The child effectively starts with a slightly dorsiflexed foot. Then I have the child stand up.

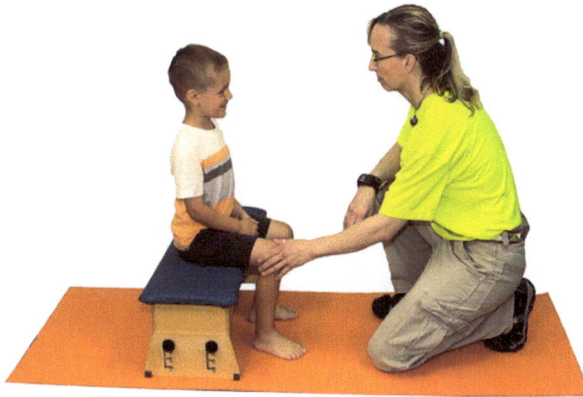

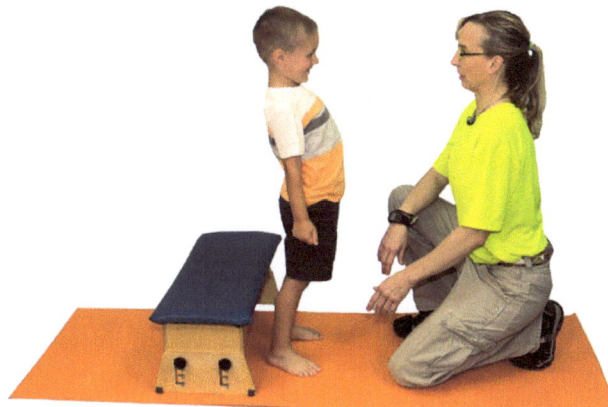

3. LOW SIT TO STAND

This exercise encourages more all-round muscle activation. Sitting lower on the bench means more hip flexion, more knee flexion, and more dorsiflexion in the starting position. This, in turn, means more hip extension, knee extension, and plantarflexion in the movement to stand up. Give the support needed for the child to be successful.

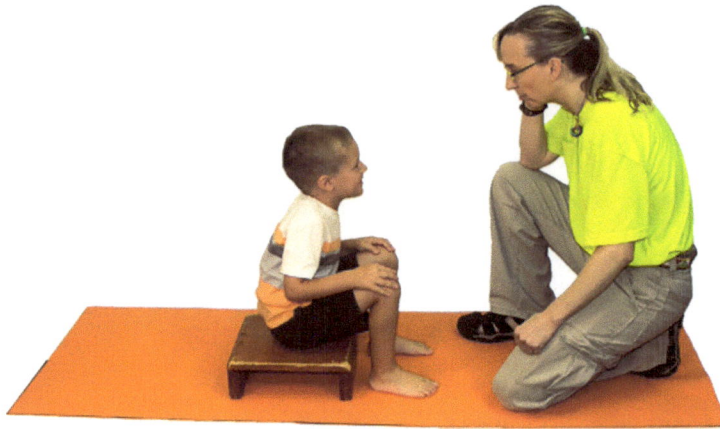

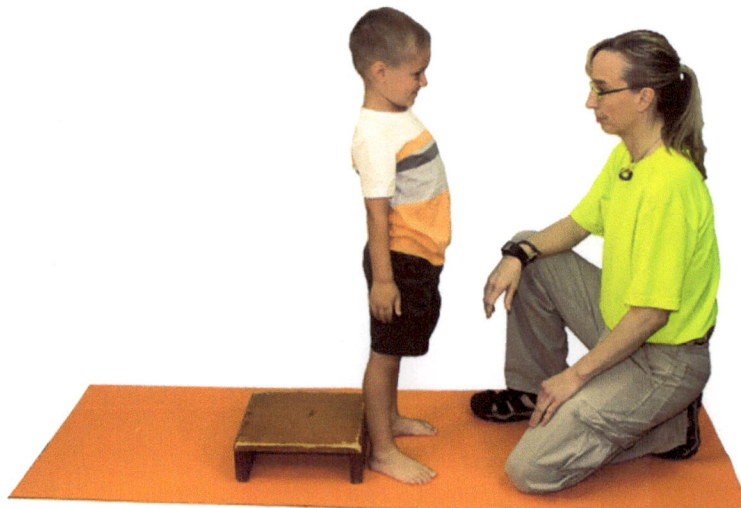

4. SQUAT TO STAND

Squat to stand works hip extensors, quadriceps, and plantarflexors, concentrically on the way up and eccentrically on the way down. I've gotten so now I try to get children to look up as they transition up and down to try to keep an arch in the back. When I am working plantarflexors, I try to get my client to put her heels down. If she has trouble, I let her stand on a decline. Or, I have her stand with her heels on a mat and her toes on the floor. Sometimes I assist with one or two hands held. Sometimes I support at the knees from the front. Or by sitting on a bench behind her, I support the knees from the back.

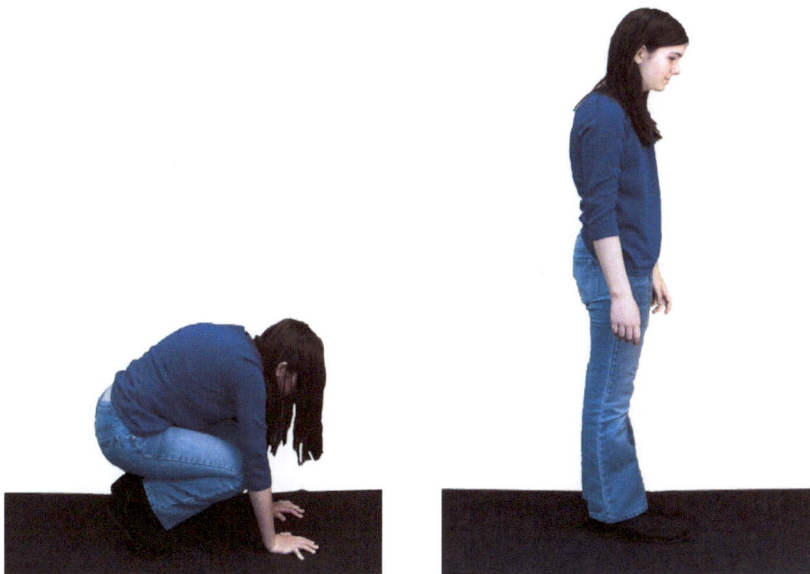

5. PUSH YOU ON A SCOOTERBOARD

Ok, I am the one that loves this activity. I finally get to go for the ride! I ride on the scooterboard, or I may use a rolling desk chair (which is definitely harder to steer, but a challenge can be a good thing). Remember that hard floors like wood or vinyl tile are much easier than pushing me on the carpet. If there is a sibling in the room, I usually let my client push the sibling. A mother or a father is fun to push too, but often the parent needs to help by pulling some with their legs. I usually motivate the child by putting stacked blocks at the finish line. The person riding knocks down the blocks dramatically and with flare. What kids like best about this activity is when I return the favor and push the child for an equal distance. I have to admit I usually start off giving the child a ride, and then I take my turn.

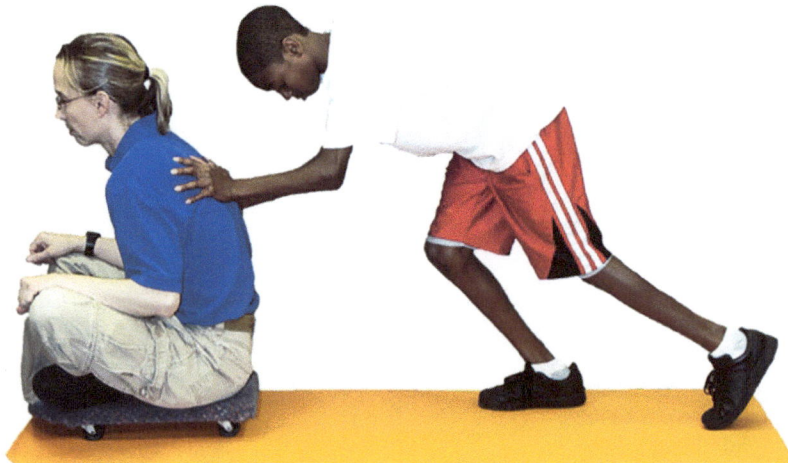

6. TIPTOES WITH ARM SUPPORT

This is one of the first ways I work on plantarflexion. In this picture,
I am allowing my model to hold onto a horizontal surface to help her
get on tiptoes. This activity becomes harder if I have her at the wall
or a mirror where she cannot assist her upward movement by pulling
down on something with her arms. Any toy with pieces works for
the activity when performed as pictured. If I am doing this activity at
the wall, then I tend to have children reach for those cling "stickers."
I like to set up the exercise so that the child actually has to move
up vertically to touch or grab something when she goes up on her
tiptoes. So many kids have trouble with plantarflexion. Instead, they
substitute with knee flexion or by rocking forward at the hips. These
substitutions will bring the heel up passively but will not achieve active
plantarflexion.

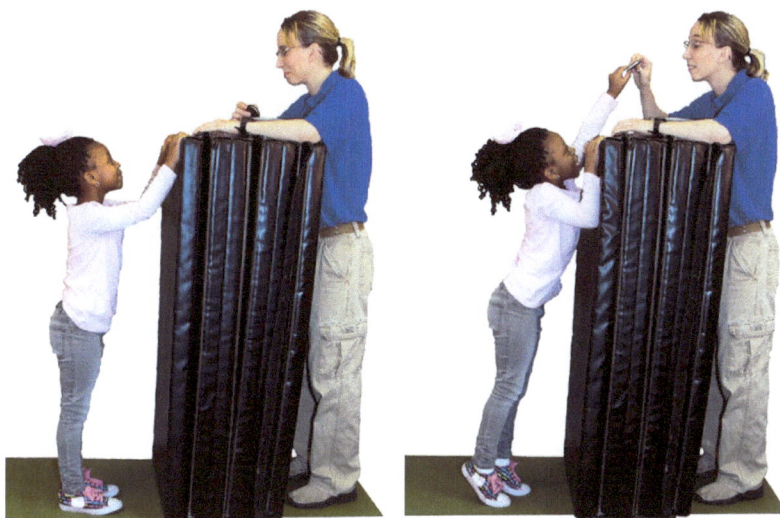

7. ONE FOOT TIPTOE WITH ARM SUPPORT

This activity is twice as hard as the previous activity by being on 1 foot instead of two. My model performs this with ease, but many of my clients have a hard time.

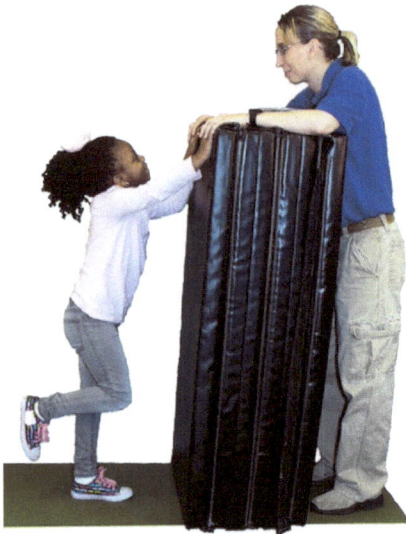

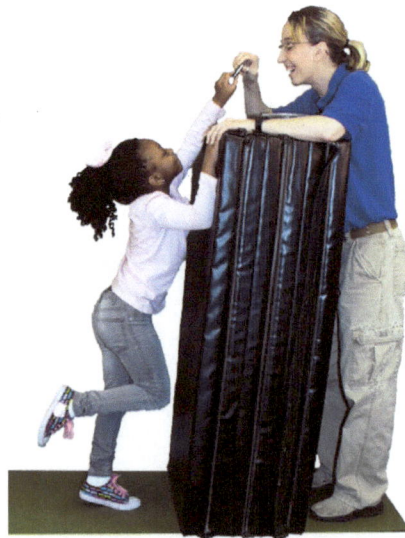

8. BILATERAL TIPTOE REACH HANDS FREE

This is an easy way to achieve plantarflexion. Just hold something up that the child wants overhead and voila! Actually, it is a little harder. I have a hard time figuring out exactly how high to put the toy to require tiptoes but not too high for the child to reach. That is why I usually prefer to put the toy on a wall or a high support. Once I figure out the right height, it is easier to duplicate. To perform the exercise as I have it pictured here, I often need a parent to tell me when I have the toy at the right height and if the child went on tiptoes or not. If I only have the toy in one hand, as in this picture, I tend to notice the child goes higher on the foot on the side she is reaching. To fix this, I usually get something like a ball that would require two hands to hold.

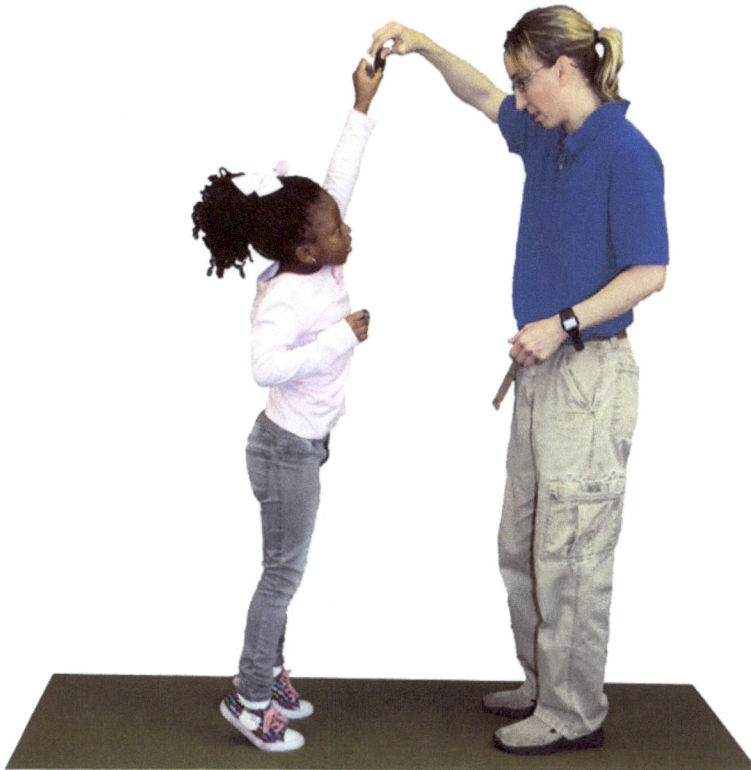

9. ONE FOOT TIPTOE REACH

Here I have the child hold onto a Kaye Products Upright Pole for support. Anything would do. I have ropes that hang down from the ceiling in my room. One of those would work well too. So would a doorknob, a wall grip, or a hand held.

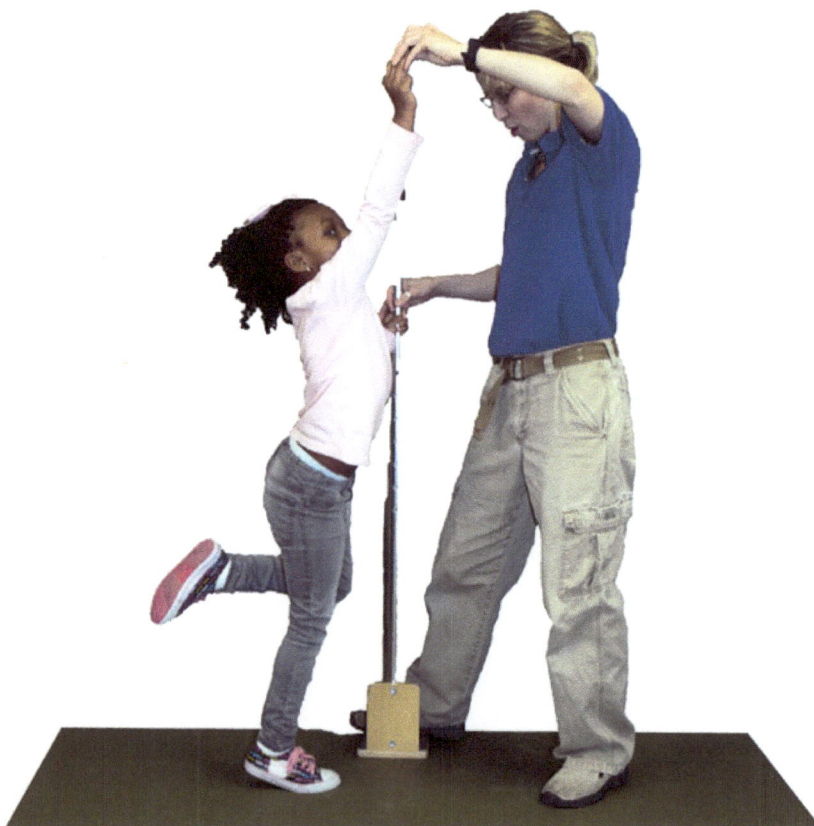

10. TIPTOE WALK

This sounds easy enough, but it isn't. Many kids have trouble figuring out how to motor plan this activity. Even when I demonstrate tiptoe walking, some kids have difficulty knowing where to look (i.e. at my feet) to understand what is the relevant part of the demonstration. If I get the parent to demonstrate, it tends to work better, especially with shoes off. Sometimes it gets comical. I may try physically to assist the child with tiptoe walking if the demonstration doesn't work. In this case, I lift the child from the armpits. My most successful trick to get a child to tiptoe walk on request is to hold a ball over her head and say, "Get it!" If a child is capable, nine times out of 10, this will work. For this little girl, I asked her to walk like a ballerina. Worked like a charm.

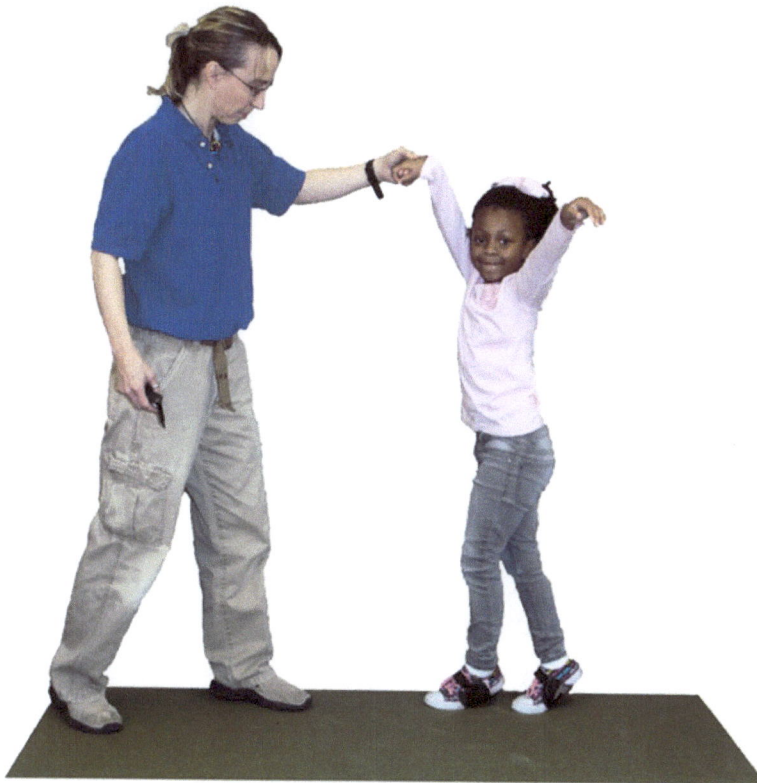

11. TIPTOES FROM A BOARD

Here, I have the child put the front of her feet up on a board. Or, I may have the front of the feet on the edge of a step or bench. If the child has no motor planning difficulties and is very cooperative, then I'll have the child perform ten reps with weight-bearing centered over the feet, then ten with the child's weight shifted to the inside of the feet, and then ten with the child's weight shift to the outside of the feet. It sounds like a subtle difference, but the weight shift significantly changes the area of muscle activation in the plantarflexors. So many kids who have trouble with plantarflexion, substitute with knee flexion or by rocking forward at the hips. These substitutions will bring the heel up passively but will not achieve active plantarflexion.

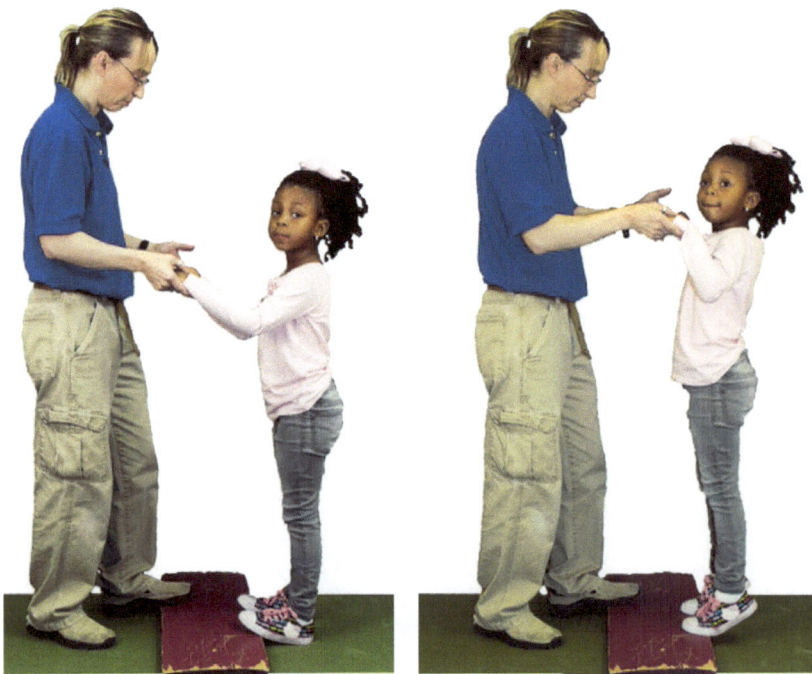

12. ONE FOOT TIPTOE FROM A BOARD

This exercise is twice as hard as the previous one. Now the child has to lift her entire body weight with one leg, not two. Here I am holding two hands, but you could also have her hold onto a wall grip or put her hands on a wall or mirror. One hand support is also an option.

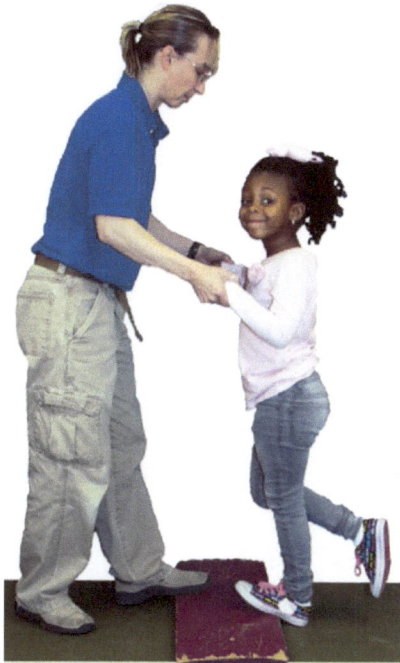

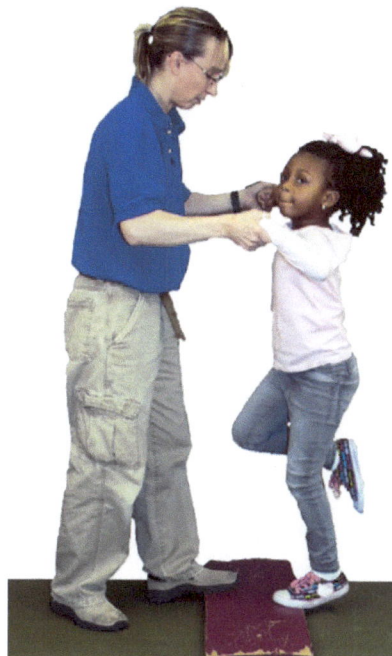

13. JUMPING UP OR OVER

I start low and work my way taller. The taller or the wider the hurdle is, the harder the hurdle is to traverse. If I go taller than 4 inches (10 cm), I have the child jump over a rope to protect the child's shins. I hold one end of the rope using a ruler for the correct height. I drape the other end of the rope over a bench on the other side. I emphasize a 2-foot take-off and landing. Many of my children have a stronger leg and lead with the weaker leg.

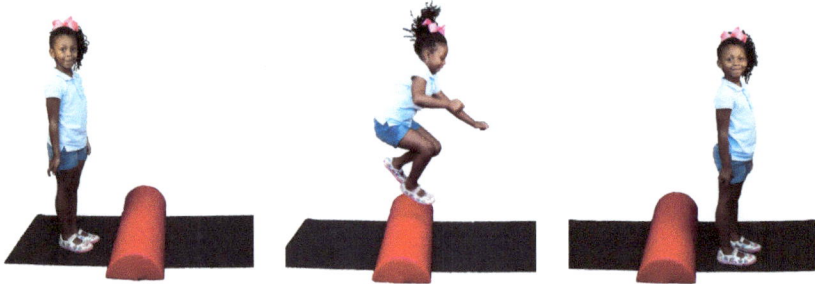

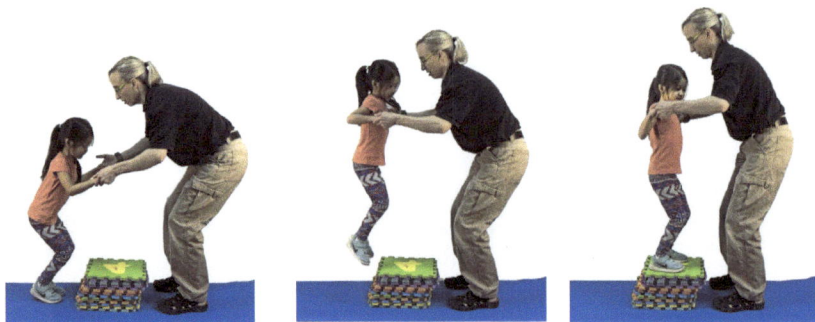

14. WALL SITS

Wall sits are primarily thought of as a glut and quad exercise, but plantarflexors are working really hard here too. I go for repetitions or duration held. I do the exercise along with the child if I think she won't fall. If I think the child might collapse, I sit on the floor in front of the child facing the child. I put up my hands up and ask the child to dip down until she touches me with her knees. This also puts me in a position to catch the child if she loses control. Work the range your child can safely control, even if that is a small movement.

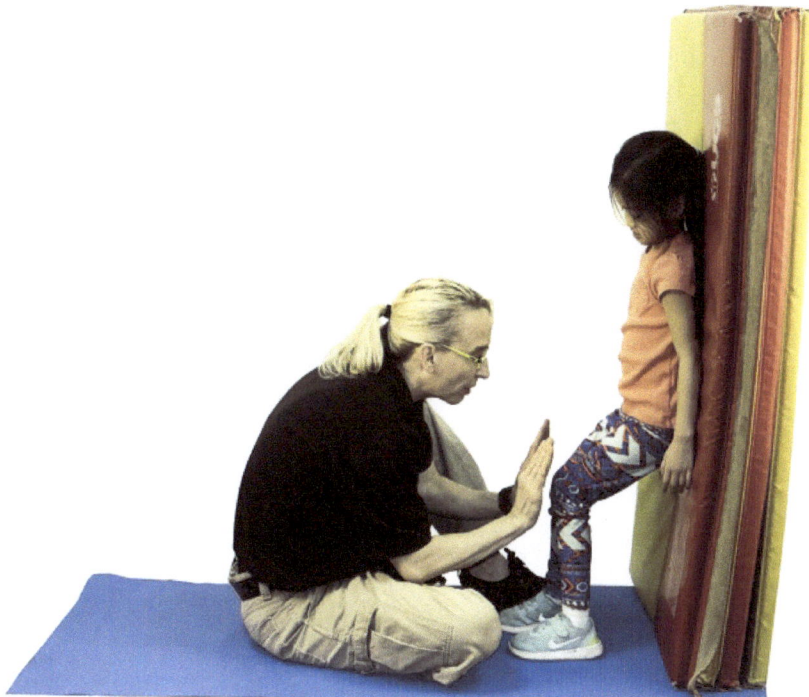

15. HOPPING ONE FOOT ON A BENCH

This plantarflexion strengthening exercise is a great first step in learning to hop on one foot. The child hops off the foot on the floor, allowing a little cheat with the foot up on the bench. Many of my children with significant weakness on one side, such as clients with hemiplegia, cheat a lot. If the leg on the floor is quite weak, the child weight shifts to the stronger leg on the bench for the lift off. In this case, I facilitate the weight shift back to the leg on the floor by holding hands. The taller the bench, the harder the leg on the ground is working. I usually don't use a bench that is higher than the child's knee. I work toward 10 hops performed consecutively without pausing. Note: The child hopping in these photos is exaggerating the hop to catch it on camera.

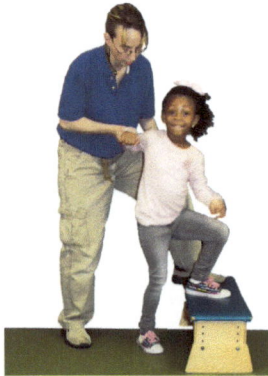

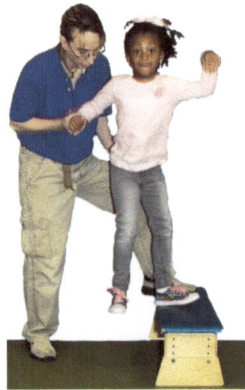

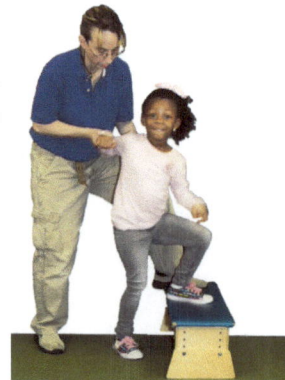

16. HOP WITH TWO HANDS ON A BENCH

Yet another plantarflexion exercise that teaches a child to hop on one foot. This one allows the child to take weight on her arms. The higher the bench, the less assistance it provides. Again, my goal is ten hops consecutively without pausing. To help, I often support the raised leg with my hand. Note: The child pictured is exaggerating the hop again.

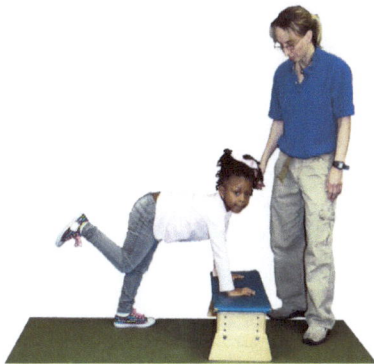

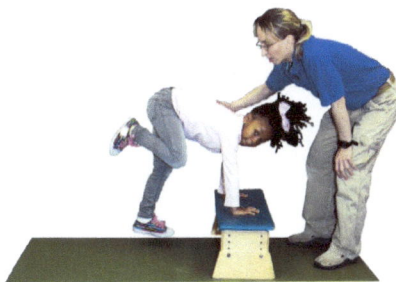

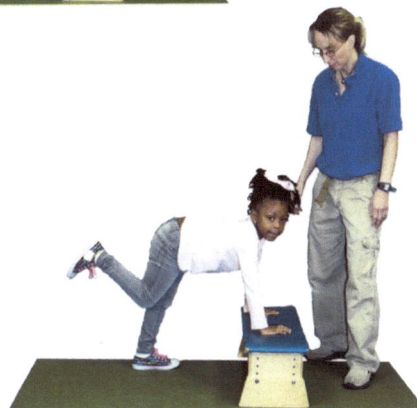

17. HOP, ONE FOOT ON A SCOOTERBOARD

This is a nice hopping on one foot exercise. By having one foot on a scooterboard (as opposed to a bench), the child is limited in how hard she can cheat with the foot on the scooterboard. Especially if the scooterboard is on hard floor such as vinyl tile, the scooterboard will just scoot away if the child pushes too hard on it.

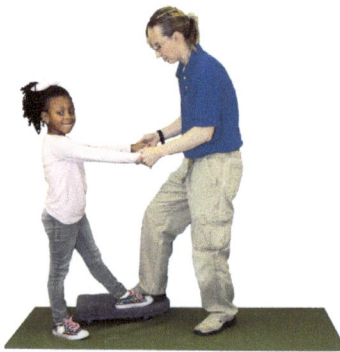

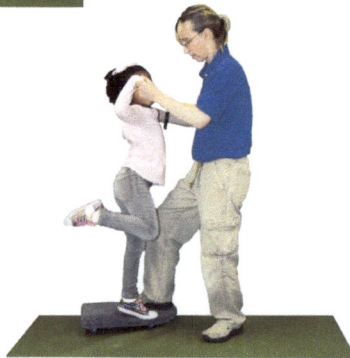

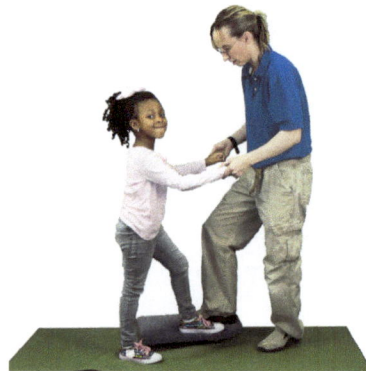

18. HOP FORWARD, ONE FOOT ON A BOARD

Set this up with the 2x4 board placed so that the 2" wide base is on the ground. Now the board easily flips over if the child cheats with the leg on the board too much. The child hops, as opposed to steps, forward, gently sliding the other foot along the board.

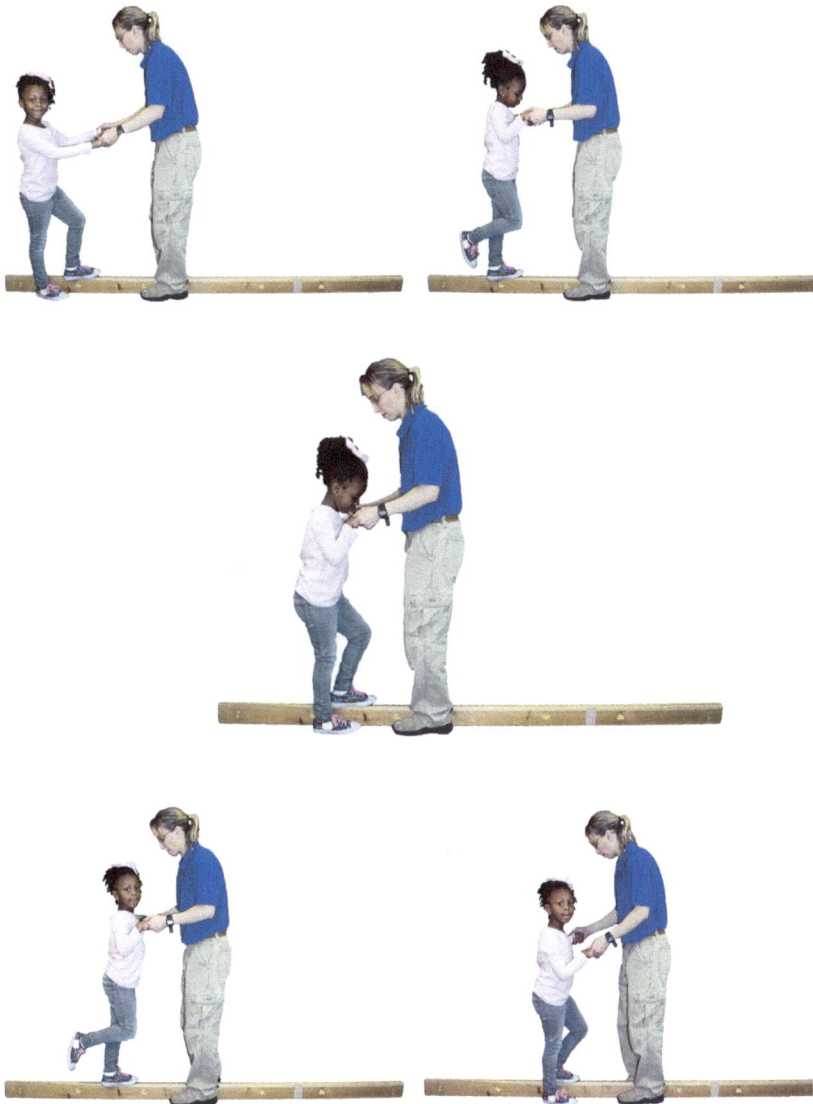

19. LAME DOG

I can usually get children to do this once, and then they remember how hard it was. Have the child hop forward with her hands on the floor and one back leg like a dog with a hurt back leg. The back leg is flexed, setting the child up for an excellent plantarflexor workout. So I don't seem like a tyrant, I do this exercise with my clients. We have a long hall at work. We lame dog down the hall, take a rest, and lame dog back.

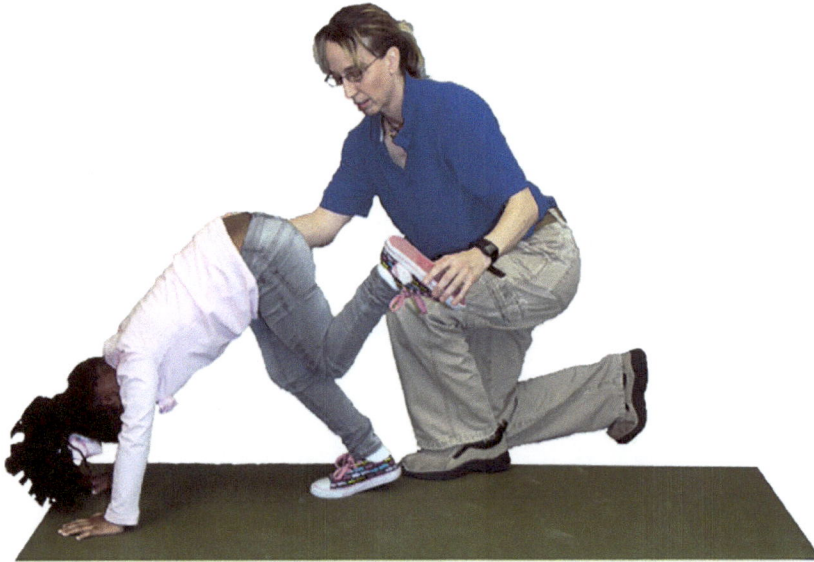

20. HOPPING ON ONE FOOT

I typically start hopping with two hands on a bench in front of a child, then two hands held, then one hand held, then two hands on the wall, then one hand on the wall, then independently. Note: The pictured hop is purposely exaggerated.

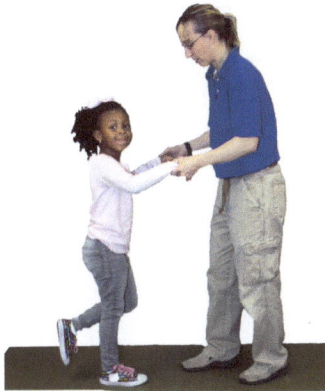

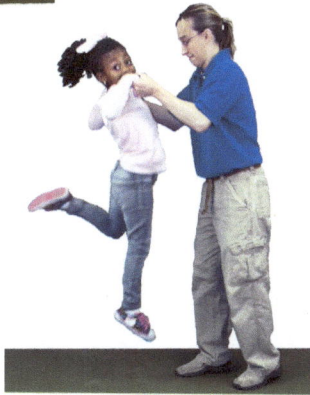

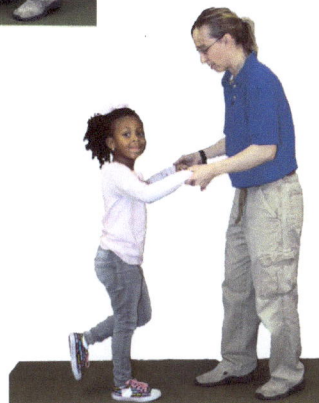

21. HOP FORWARD

New hoppers tend to hop in place or in a circle. Hopping forward requires more dorsiflexion range and ankle control. I help the child hop forward with two or one hand held or independently. I like to have a child hop forward down the hall with one hand on the wall. Hopping with the foot up closest to the wall is easier with its wider base of support. To make it harder, pick up the furthest foot from the wall. When the child uses the wall as a support, I can help hold the child's free hand or hold up the raised foot.

To challenge balance and strength, have the child hop forward to consecutive carpet squares, balancing on each for a three count, before hopping to the next. Start with the carpet squares close and work progressively wider.

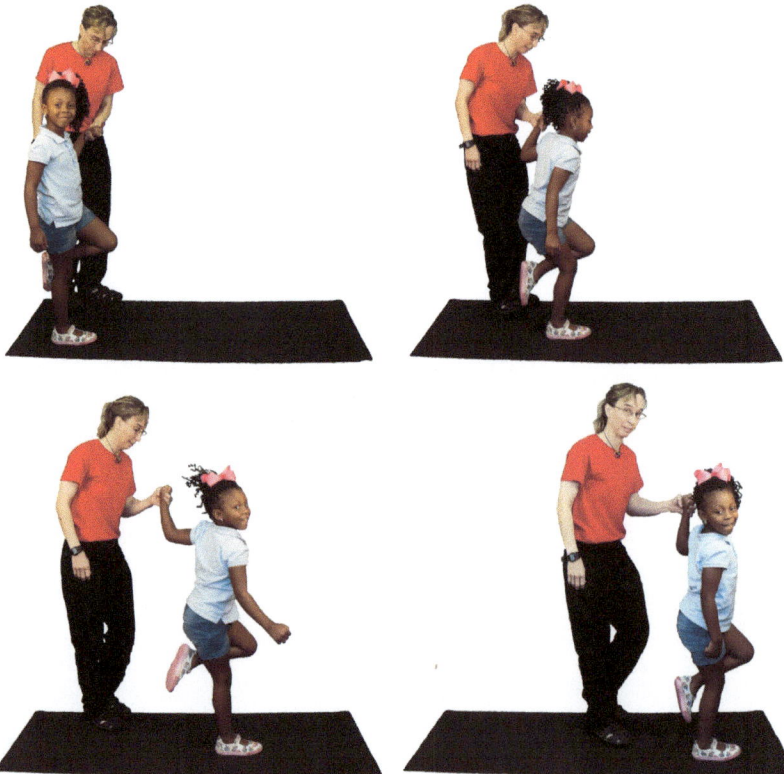

22. HOP FORWARD ON A LINE

For my advanced hoppers, I have them hop on one foot forward on a
line. At the clinic, I put hook Velcro down to make lines on our carpet.
I put two rows down to make the line twice as wide. Staying on the
line requires significantly more control.

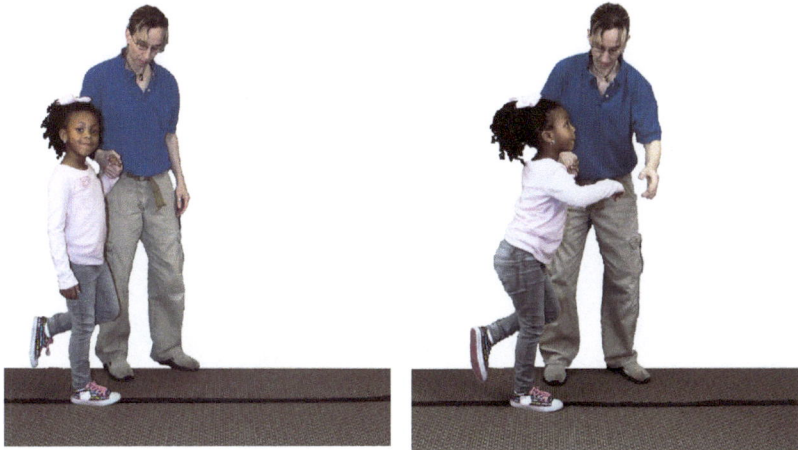

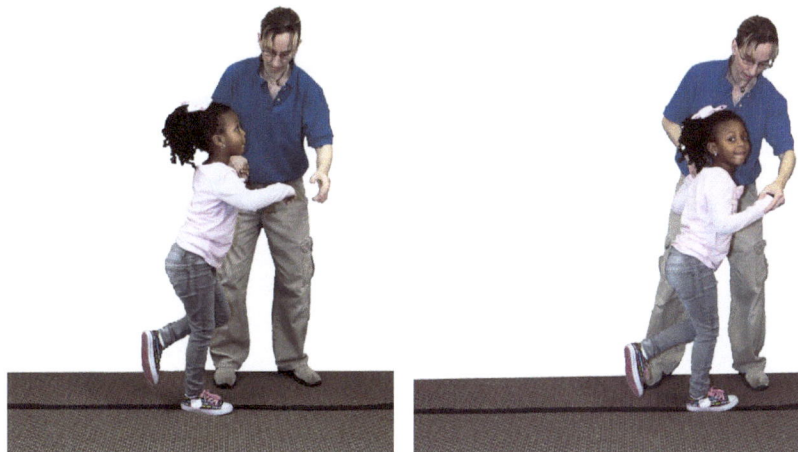

23. HOP UP THE STAIRS

Oh, this is a challenging exercise. I usually make sure the child can hop on one foot with support onto folded mats before going to the stairs. Folded mats are more forgiving than stairs. Hitting your shin on the stairs really hurts. I start holding a child's hand and having her hold the rail on the other side. Some children are big enough to hold the railing on both sides of the stairs. After a child can hop on one foot up the stairs with two hand support, I progress to one hand support.

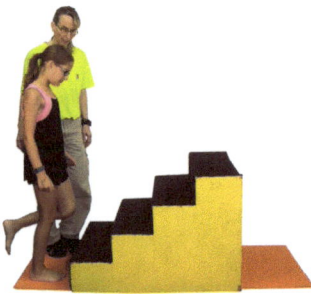

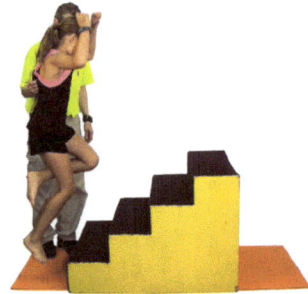

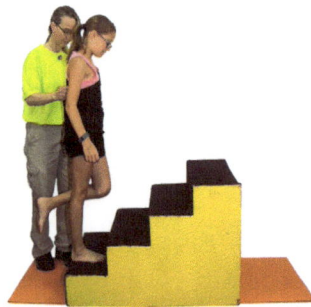

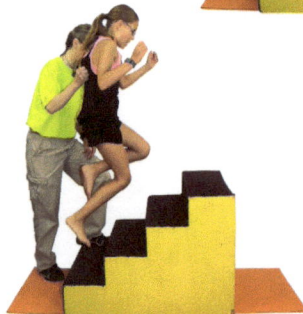

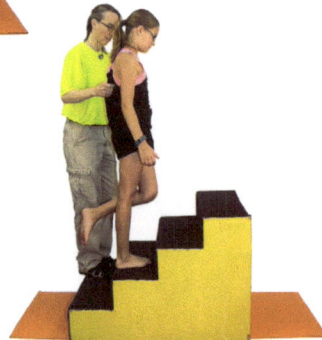

24. DON'T SQUEAK--TALL BENCH

I have many clients who need to work on control of plantarflexion/
knee extension/hip extension. I love this exercise for midrange control
of gluts, quads, and plantarflexors. Without control, if he bends too
much, he collapses down. I have the client stand in front of a bench
with a squeak toy or piano on it. He is to stoop down and touch the
piano or squeak toy with his bottom--but not squeak it. Obviously,
this is much easier if you don't have to go down too low. I love the
Kaye Products adjustable benches that allow you to modify the
benches height one inch at a time until you find the right height for
the perfect challenge for the client. I love sound effects and so do my
clients. This exercise is usually fun. If the client faces a mirror, it is
easier for him to see the squeak toy's distance.

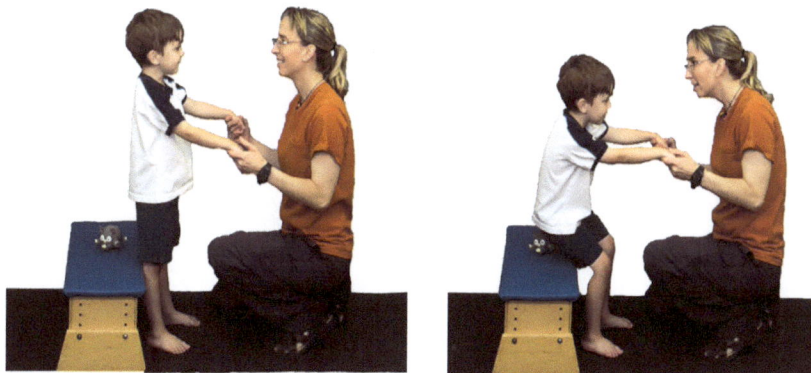

25. DON'T SQUEAK--SMALL BENCH

Just an inch lower makes this activity potentially much harder. If you don't have an adjustable bench, you can always make the bench an inch shorter by putting a single thickness mat under the client's feet, but not under the bench. The bench just became effectively shorter. You can continue along the same lines by doubling and then tripling the mat.

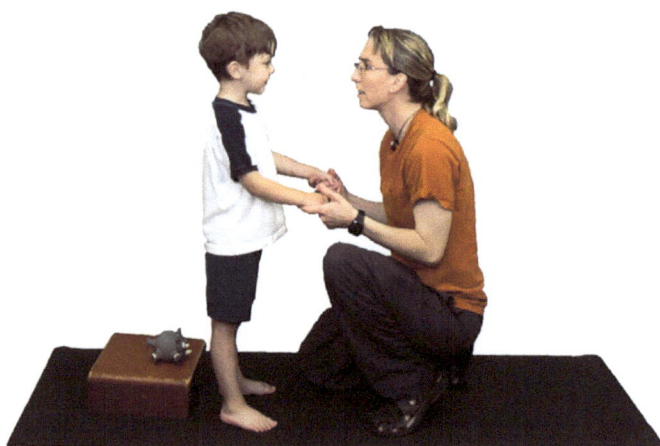

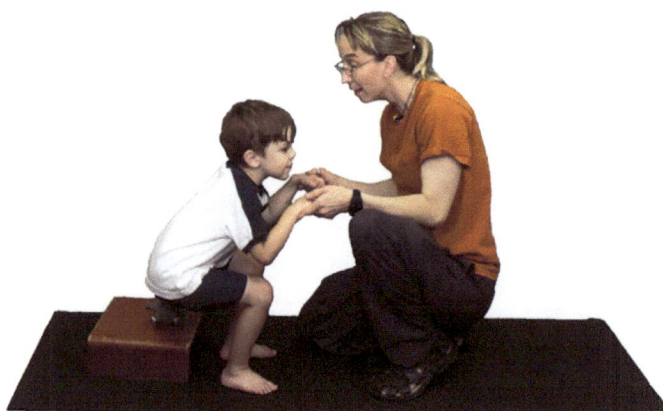

26. KNEEL TO HALF KNEEL TO STAND

Half kneel to stand is a terrific hip/knee extension and plantarflexion exercise. I work on kneel to ½ kneel to stand at furniture, at a wall, at two poles, with one pole, with one hand held, with one hand on the wall with my client facing sideways. Seems like one of the big keys is getting the weight shifted forward so the head is over the knee that is up. I facilitate this transition in this picture series without support, but probably more commonly I give knee support from the front when a client is close to performing the transition independently. Several of my kids have learned to do this transition with both hands on the raised knee. Then I fade to only one hand allowed on the raised knee and then entirely independently. I am not typically satisfied until a child can transition up and down 5-10 repetitions with either leg raised and hands free.

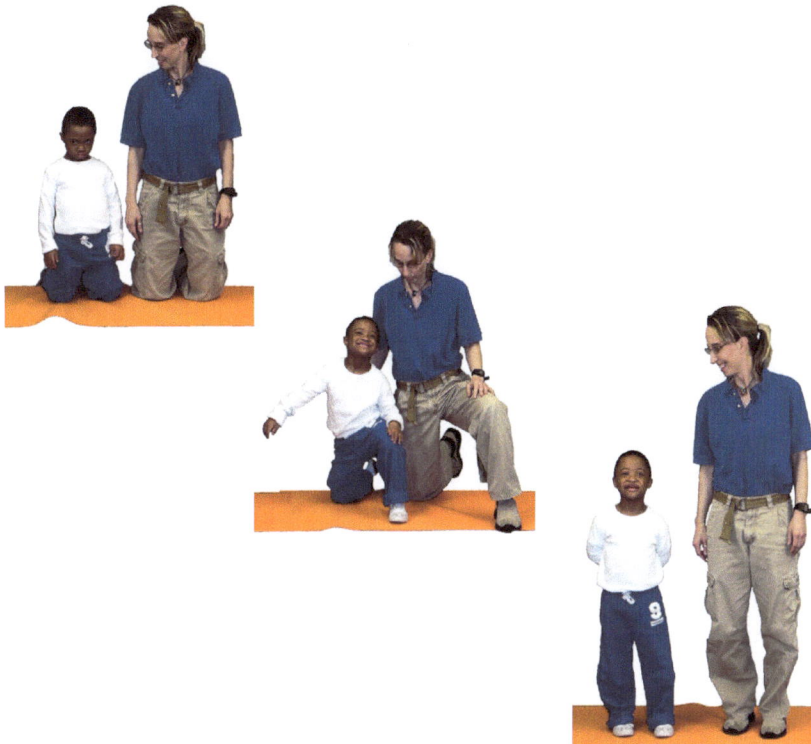

27. LUNGE TO STAND HANDS HELD

Here my model needed support mostly to get back up to standing again from the lunge position. I usually mark on my carpeted floor with Velcro lines where I want my client to start, to step out to, and to step back to in one big step. I start with small distances and work further out with success. I always try to get the child to put the non-stepping knee down to the floor. This exercise works hip and knee extensors and plantarflexors powerfully.

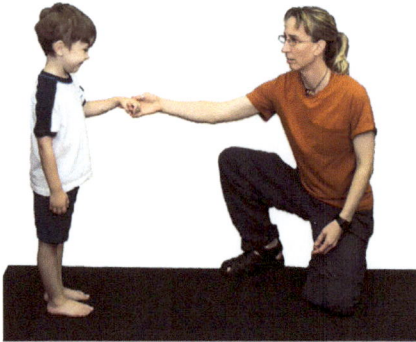

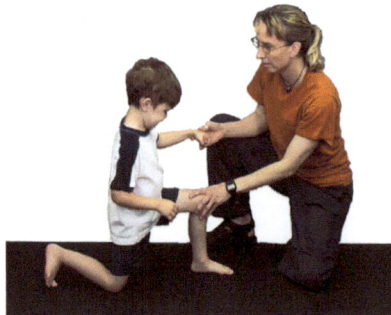

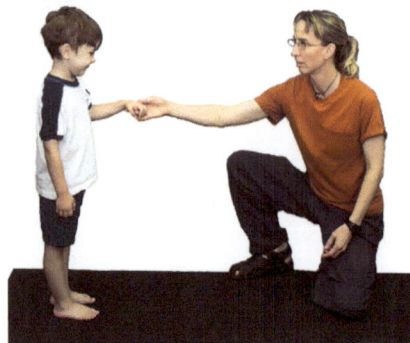

28. STAND TO HALF KNEEL

I love emphasizing both parts of the transition--the ½ kneel to stand and then the stand to ½ kneel. Most of my clients figure out the transition into standing with control before standing to ½ kneel. I frequently have to help bring back the leg for them to initiate the movement down. Controlling the descent to ½ kneel emphasizes the eccentric muscle contractions of hip/knee extensors and plantarflexors.

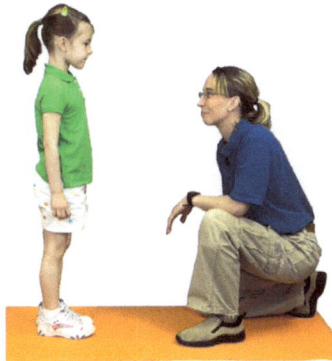

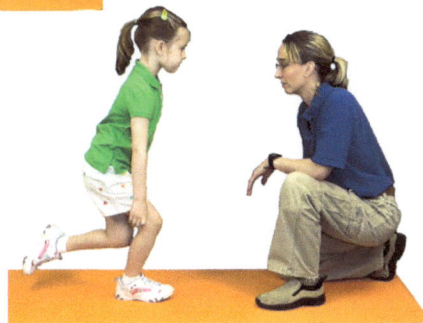

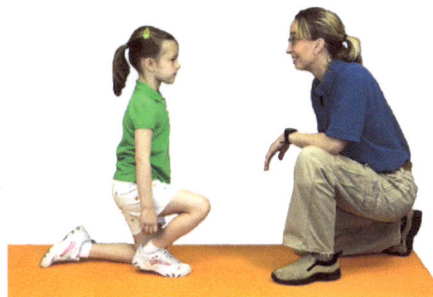

29. WALK UP STAIRS

Stair work is excellent for gluts, quads, and plantarflexors. I progress from trunk support from behind, to two hands held, to one hand on a rail and one hand held, to one hand held, to one hand on the rail, to one hand on a wall to independently. I have clients who can't walk or stand independently, but we practice the stairs. It is a terrific leg strengthening exercise. I support the child from behind and lift one leg (if she can't do it by herself) to the next step. I ask the child to push through the leading leg to ascend to the next step. Then I ask her to bring the trailing leg to the step the other foot is on--and repeat. I usually do one flight of stairs leading with the left foot and then one flight of stairs leading with the right foot. I have to remind most of my clients with cerebral palsy to lean forward "nose over toes" instead of extending dangerously backward. I also remind the child to slide her hand on the rail one to two steps ahead after each step. "Step, Slide, Step, Slide." I prefer to walk behind a client to spot them on the stairs.

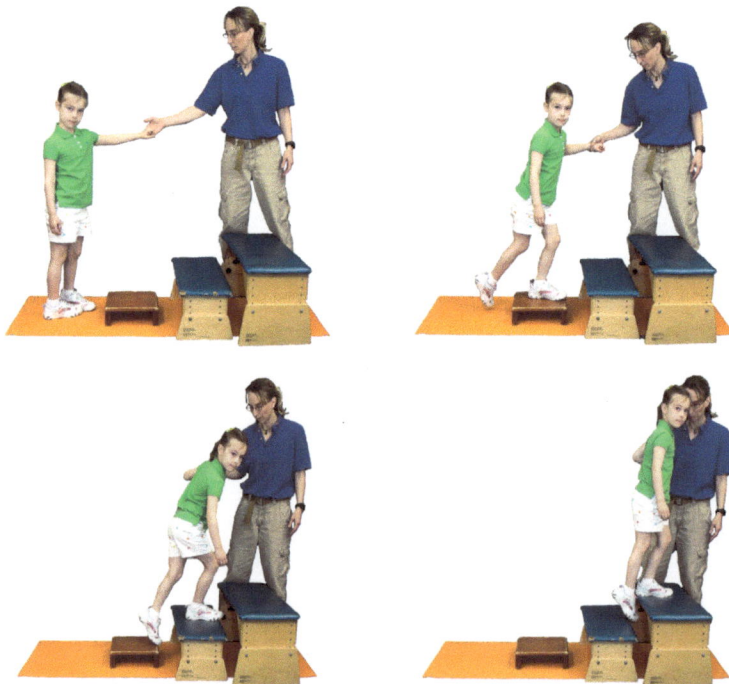

30. DOWN THE STAIRS SLOWLY

Slow downstairs work emphasizes eccentric strengthening and control of the plantarflexors, knee and hip extensors. I progress the support similar to the previous exercise. With a nonambulatory client, I support the child from behind, weight shift her to take a step, and then help to lower her to the next step. I ask her to bring the trailing leg to the step the other foot is on--and repeat. I do one flight of stairs leading with each. Going down is a lot easier than going up. This is an important skill to have for safety. If the elevator isn't working, at least you can get the child down the stairs. It is much easier to walk a child down the stairs than to deadlift a heavy child down the stairs.

I spot a less competent ambulatory client from behind. I keep my hands on a belt at the child's hips, and I am ready to pull the child back onto my lap if there is a problem. When I am confident in a child's safety, I go in front of the child to spot her. I remind clients to hold the railing in the front instead of hanging off the railing behind them.

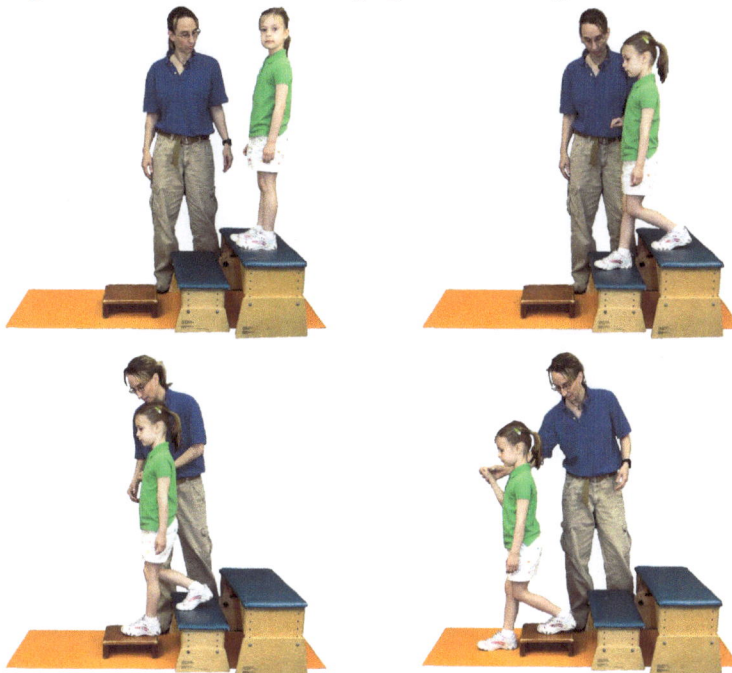

31. ONE LEG STOOP AND RECOVER

Kids tend to like or at least tolerate this game. If you don't have a pole, then a doorknob or the corner of a table works as well. For a higher-level client, I don't stabilize the pole and let her work through the instability. For the most advanced clients, I don't let my client hold the pole at all. For the rings to put on the pole, I use either the larger swimming pool rings that children dive for or rigid bracelets. Kids like the bracelets because if the child spins it just right, it will spin down the pole. If a child needs more help, I support the raised leg. I have the child lift the leg closest to the pole for a broader base of support or raise the further foot for a more significant challenge. If I put the ring forward a little further on the floor, I get a more plantarflexion movement than if the ring is close to the child's foot. This exercise is a wonderful strengthener of gluts, quads, and plantarflexors.

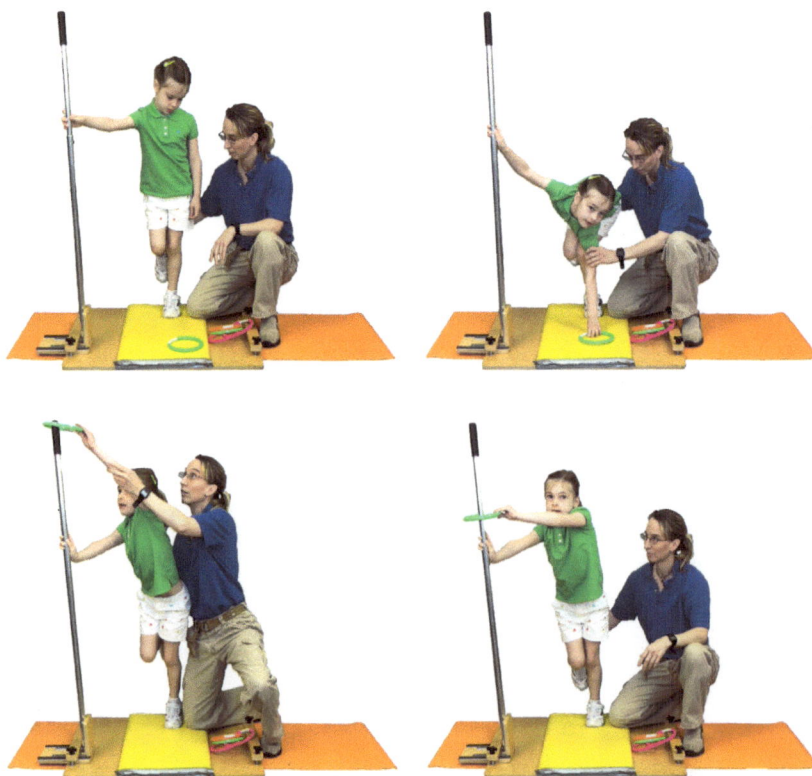

32. FOOT BACK ON BENCH PICK UP

This game doesn't win me any points as a therapist with the kids. This
activity is challenging. The taller the bench in the back, the harder this
activity is. I usually don't go any higher than the kid's knee. I remind
the child that I only want the toe on the bench--not the whole foot. I
love this activity as it works on balance and strength. You get eccentric
muscle contractions on the descent and concentric on the way up.
Toys with pieces are the key. Here the child is picking up those shape
puzzle oreo cookies. Again, I see more movement at the hip, ankle,
and knee when I put the toy further away from the child's foot.

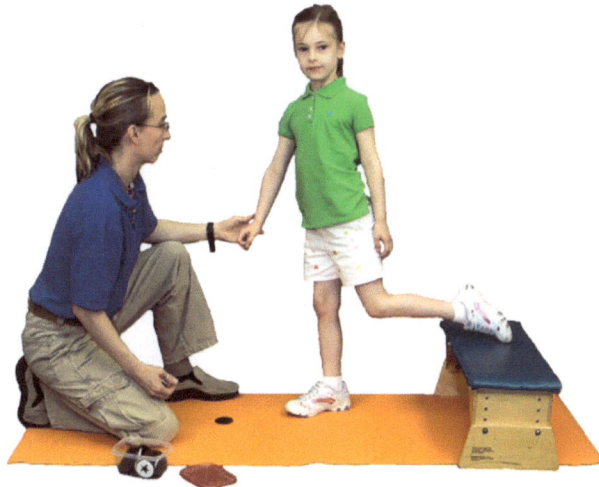

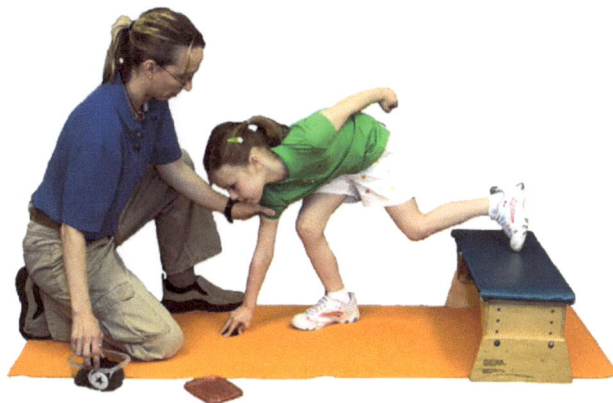

33. LOWER ONE LEG STOOP AND RECOVER

To encourage more hip/knee extension and plantarflexion strengthening, have the client pick up an object even lower. I've had a few higher level clients with hemiplegia who could perform this activity with hands free—but the majority can't get to this level or need additional assistance.

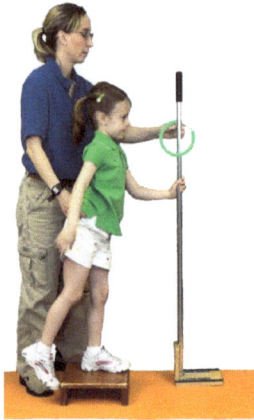

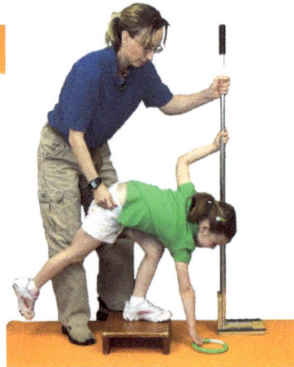

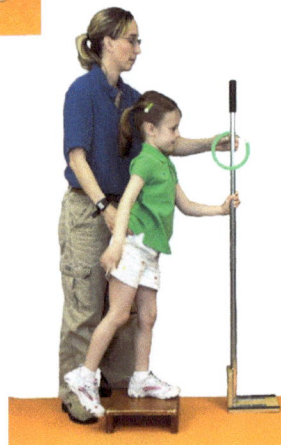

34. BACKWARD STEP UP AND DOWN

I perform this with a single bench up and down to get both the concentric and eccentric quads/gluts/plantarflexors. I have the child do the entire movement standing with his back to the bench, stepping back putting one foot and then the other on the bench. Sometimes I let the child leave one foot on the bench behind him. Then he steps the opposite leg up and down repetitively.

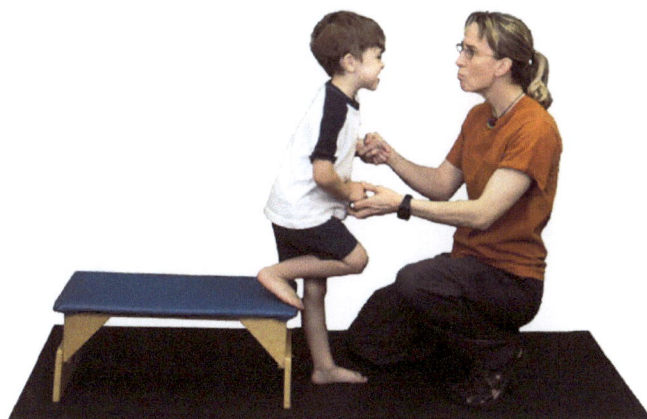

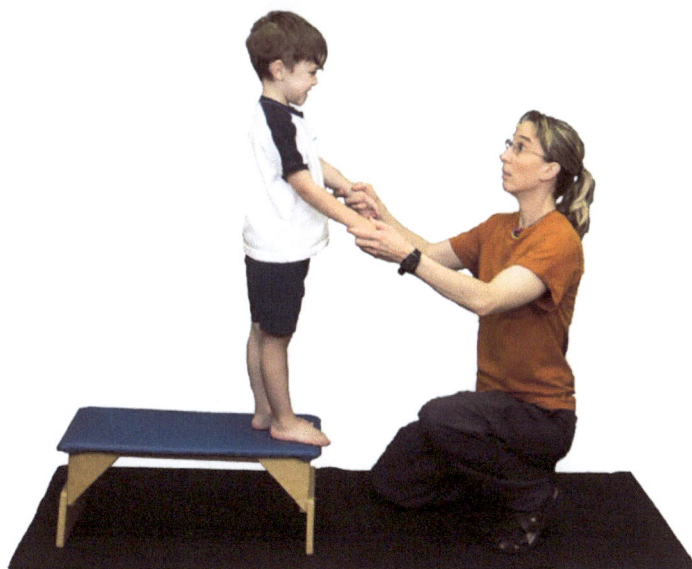

35. BACKWARD DOWN THE STAIRS

This is, of course, the complement exercise to walking backward up the stairs. Backward down the stairs emphasizes eccentric quads/gluts and plantarflexors. Honestly, I like the stairs. With the 20 steps at my facility between floors, I get 20 repetitions. Encouraging a child to do 20 reps on a bench is trickier. As needed, I progress the level of assistance from trunk support, to two hands held, to one hand on a rail and one hand held, to one hand held, to one hand on the rail, to one hand on a wall, to independently. Most kids think this is cool and don't give me a hard time with this activity.

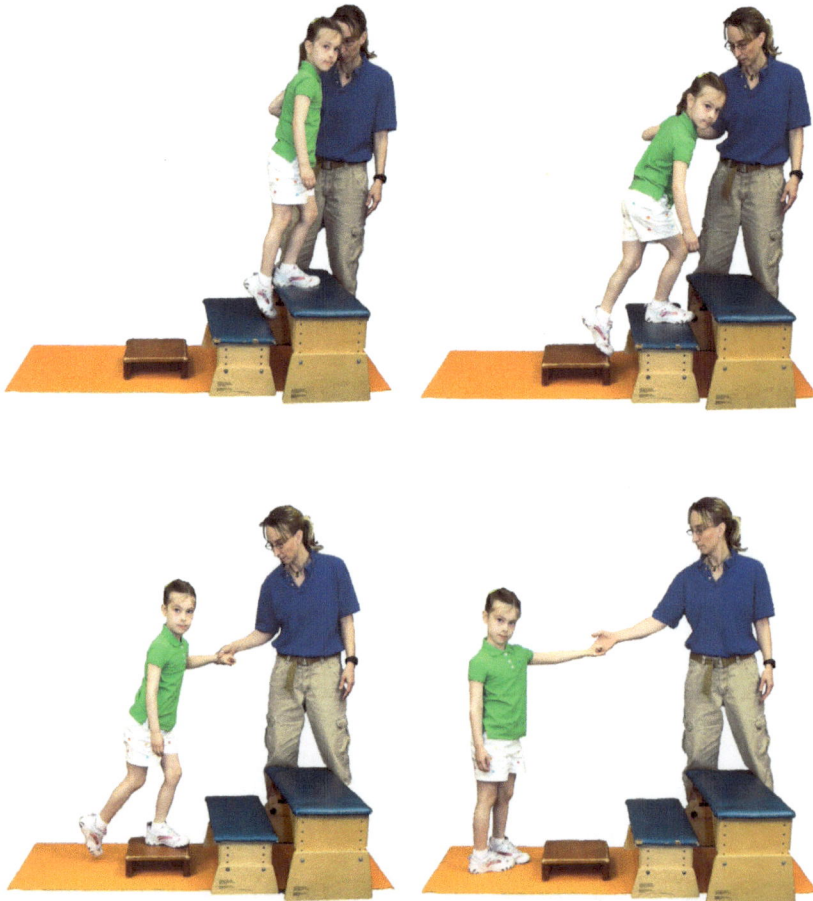

36. KNOCK DOWN BLOCKS WITH KNEES

This is a more recent favorite. This movement emphasizes eccentric plantarflexors and end range quadriceps. To progress the level of difficulty, I start with two hands held, then one hand held, then no support. I start with the blocks set up, touching the end of the child's toes. Ensure the object being knocked over is at least knee height or the exercise becomes exponentially more challenging. The child must allow the tibia to ride forward over the foot with control. This exercise is particularly tricky for toe walkers. To make it harder, I move the block away from the child's incrementally, or I try it on one leg.

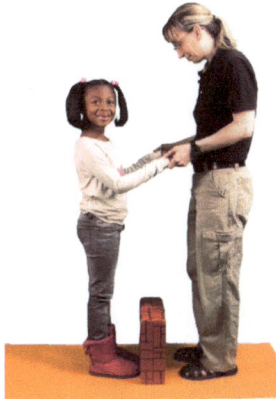

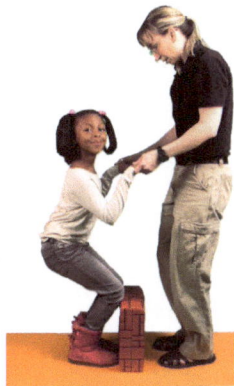

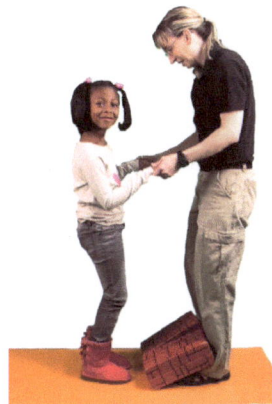

37. DIP KICKS

I prefer upright poles, but I have used one railing and a hand held
for this activity. A child of any height can hold the poles at the
right height for them. I start with two poles and then work to one.
I strategically place the pole to provide a wider or narrower base of
support with the stance leg. To make this harder, I forego the pole and
let the child put a hand on the wall. It never hurts to have a spot on
this activity. I usually am down low, placing the toy to be kicked. So I
am not in a great position to spot the child if there is a balance loss. I
have a parent stand nearby to spot.

Technically, the differential between the height of the bench and
the toy makes this more challenging. First, I make the toy lower, and
then I make the bench higher. Often a child simply plantarflexes
the kicking foot to knock over the toy. You'll have to put the toy low
enough that the child has to bend her stance hip/knee/ankle. To
maximize the difficulty, I put the bench close to the wall and ask the
child to use it only with a potential loss of balance. Or I resort to the
dreaded double, triple, quadruple, etc. dip kicks. With these, I hold
the toy, and the child must repeatedly dip down to kick the toy before
putting her foot back on the bench, all the while maintaining at least
slight knee flexion.

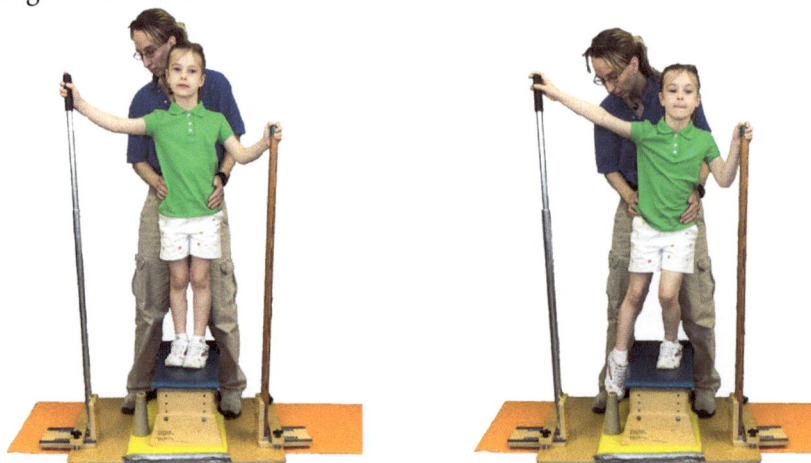

38. STAND ON A DECLINE

I was surprised how difficult this was for a child with weak plantarflexors. This exercise is for isometric plantarflexors. I use the basic heelcord stretching wedge but have the child stand on it with toes pointing down. I can hold two hands or one hand, or let the child stand independently. I distract the child from the work she is doing with games like hitting the balloon back and forth or throwing and catching a ball.

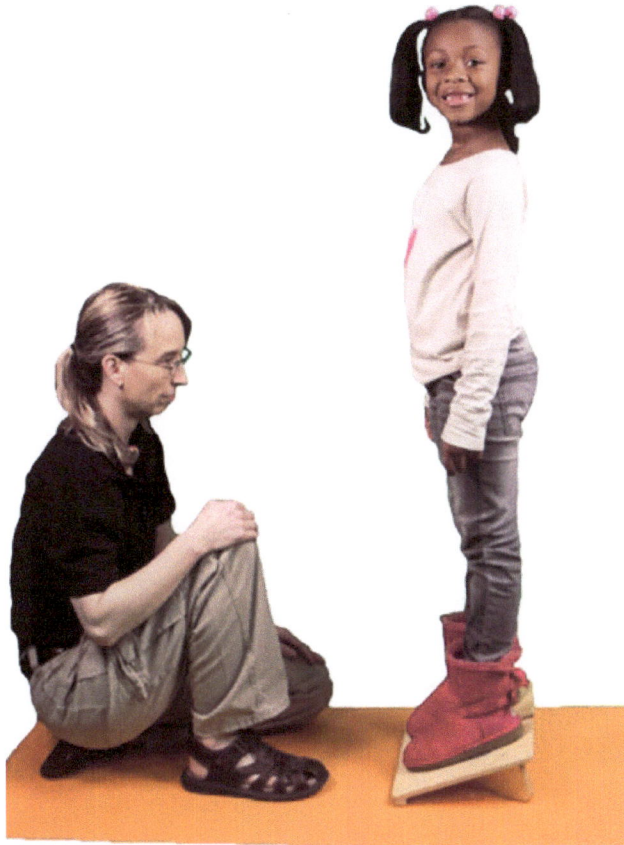

39. STAND ON A DECLINE ON ONE FOOT

Standing on one foot more than doubles the challenge. This exercise packs a balance and a strength component. Again, I can hold two hands or one hand or let the child stand independently. Playing distracting games here compounds the level of difficulty.

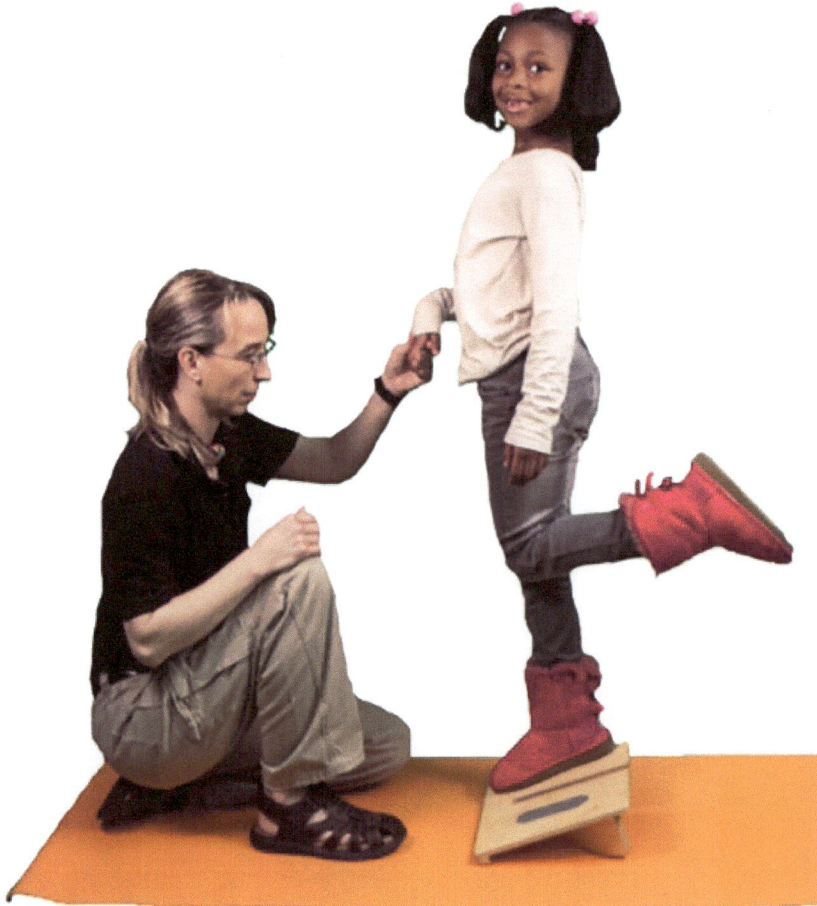

40. STANDING SCOOTERBOARD RIDING

I love this exercise. So do the kids. I have the child stand with both
feet on one scooterboard or with each foot on its own scooterboard.
It kind of reminds me of water skiing. I pull my kids around the clinic,
holding their hands. This is deceptively hard. It is particularly tough
to control on smooth flooring and easier on the carpeting at the clinic.
The transitions between the two different surfaces are very tricky. You
might want to have another adult/parent spot for safety. Watch out
for your low shins. Successful riding requires a very delicate balance of
strength in plantarflexion and dorsiflexion.

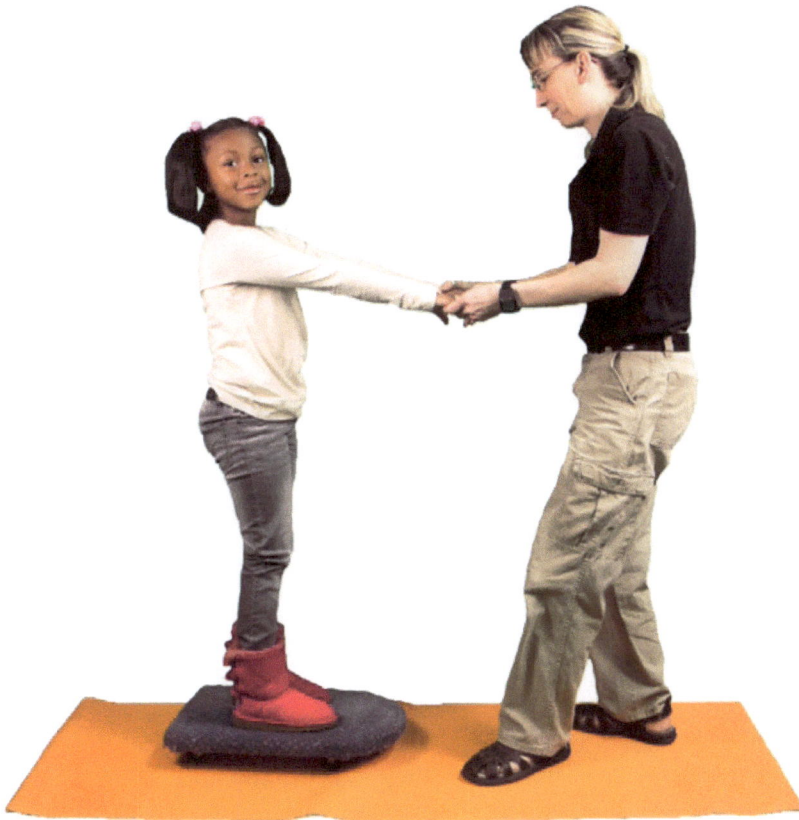

41. SCOOTERBOARD RIDING ON ONE LEG

This is more than twice as hard! Make sure the child has mastered the two-legged version before progressing to one leg.

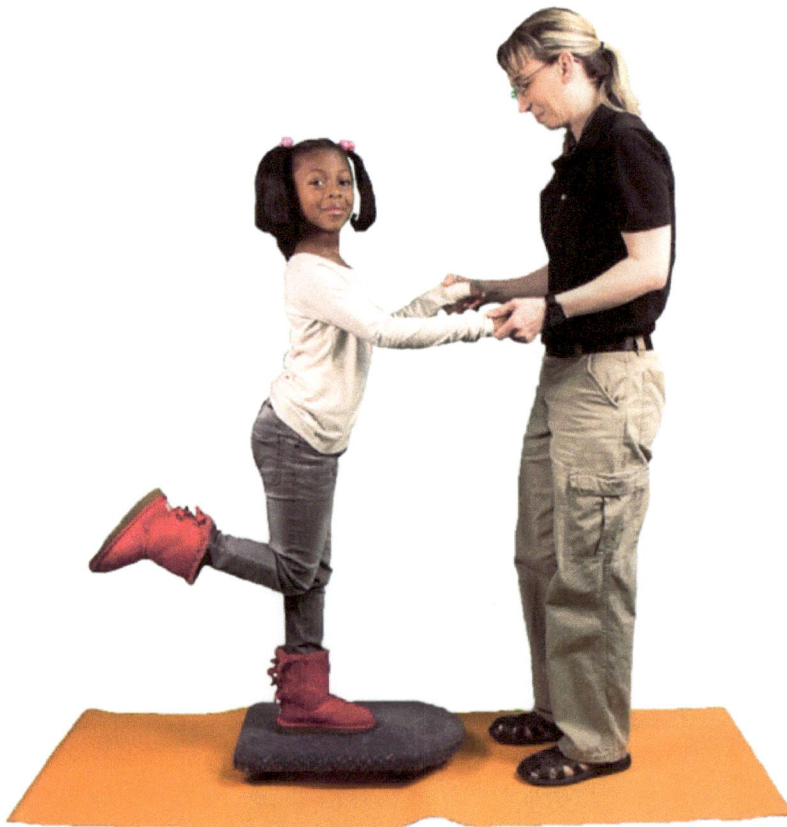

42. SOLEUS SCOOTERBOARD RIDE

This recent addition to my repertoire targets the soleus muscle group by getting tiptoes work with knee flexion. Have the child take short steps keeping the feet close up under the knees to encourage more soleus pushing forward and less hamstring pulling forward work.

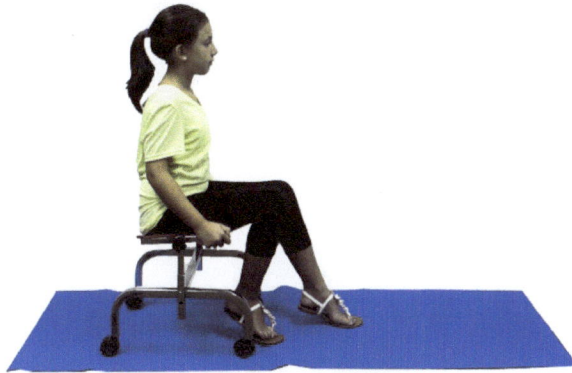

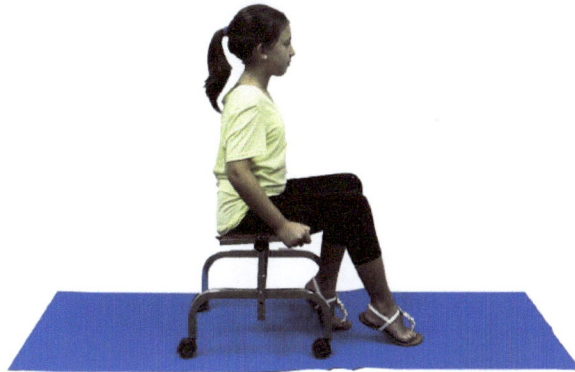

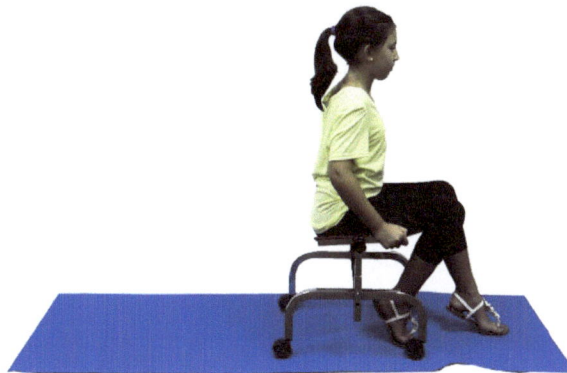

II. DORSIFLEXION

THE ANKLE DORSIFLEXORS PULL THE top of the foot toward the shin. Activating your dorsiflexors makes you stand on your heels or pull up your foot. Weakness in the dorsiflexors make it difficult to lift the foot for running or walking. As pediatric physical therapists, we often deal with weakness in the dorsiflexor group associated with cerebral palsy or toe walking. This chapter includes a wide variety of exercises to improve ankle dorsiflexion strength and control.

* * *

1. WALK UP AN INCLINE OR HILL

This is one of the easiest dorsiflexion exercises. By having a child walk up a natural or manufactured incline, dorsiflexion is encouraged. Watch for substitutions of hip flexion or out-toeing. The steeper the pitch, the more dorsiflexion is likely required. I usually encourage a heel toe gait, but with some of my toe walkers, I may simply try to get the heel down at all. Some children can't start on an incline and need to start on the flat floor. For my toe walkers, I remind the child that it is a little easier to get the heel to touch down with longer stride lengths. I can use an angle finder on the incline to get an idea of the angle of inclination for documentation purposes. I can have the child walk independently, with two hands held, one hand held, or a walker. I document the gait pattern, the number of correct steps, or the duration walked with the appropriate form.

For a never-ending incline, a treadmill works great. I like a treadmill because I can position myself low beside the child and watch to see if the heel is hitting before the toe (or if the heel is making contact at all). I can modify the speed, duration, support required, and the incline angle. Spot your child closely for safety and use the safety tether if available.

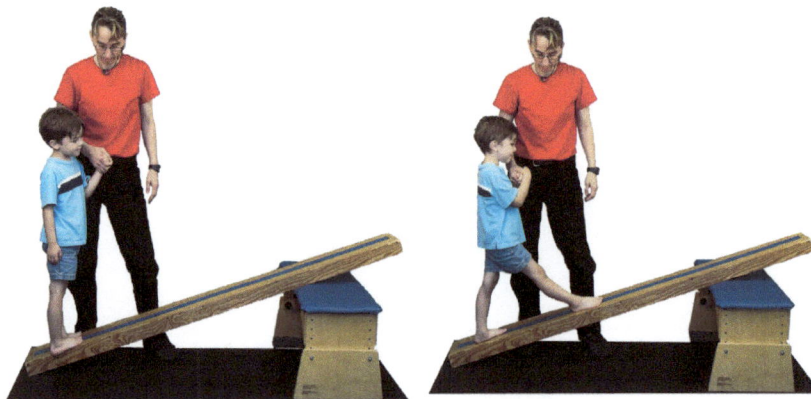

2. CLIMBING

Most children, except the gravitationally insecure, love to climb. I have an angle-adjustable climbing wall at the clinic that I love. So do the kids. Climbing does not require dorsiflexion, but it sure makes it easier.

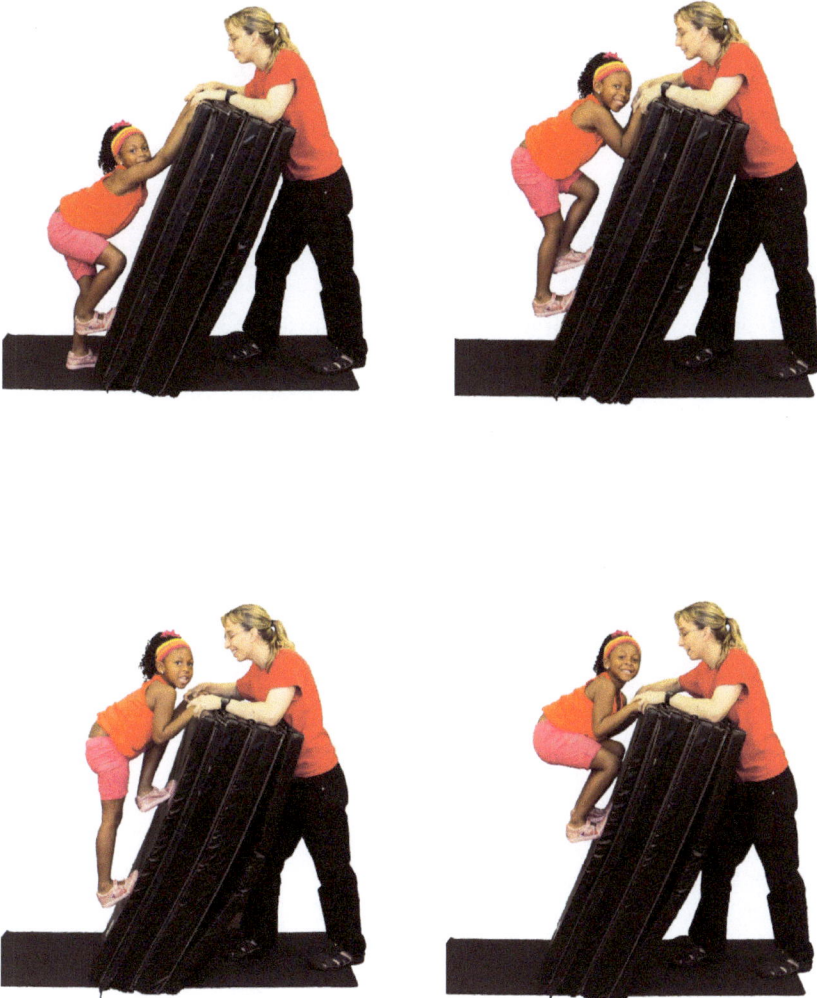

3. MANUAL RESISTANCE DORSIFLEXION

In this position, I hold the child's lower calf between my knees and discourage cheating. I use one hand to provide resistance/assistance to the foot and the other hand as the target. I tend to position the target hand by having my pinky on the shin. The child touches my thumb with his foot. This way, wherever the shin goes, my target hand moves along with it. Children try to scoot back in their chair to bring the foot up. This way of providing the target eliminates the effectiveness of that cheat. The target position is essential. Usually, a child has more passive range than active, so don't put the target position in an impossible to reach position--unless you plan to assist significantly at the end of the range. Some children cannot for the life of them motor plan how to pull the foot up. I resort to a little bottom of the foot tickle to see if it will jerk up into dorsiflexion. Or I use electric stimulation to help a child get the feeling of dorsiflexion.

I perform this activity concentrically, but also eccentrically. I allow the child to dorsiflex his foot, and I try to pull it down to a target--usually my shirt. If I pull his foot down to my shirt before I get to the count of 10, I win. Children are amazingly motivated to win a competition with their therapist.

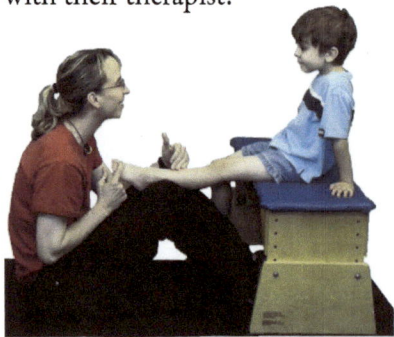

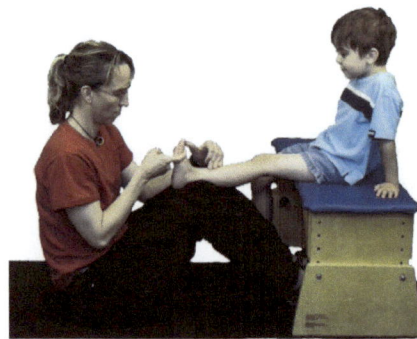

4. ROCKING FORWARD/BACK

Don't forget righting reactions extend down to the feet. It is worth
trying rocker board work to see if you can get some dorsiflexion
activation with balance reactions with anterior/posterior tilting.

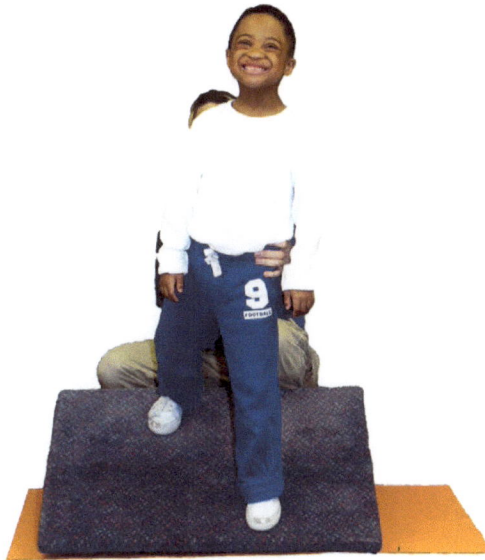

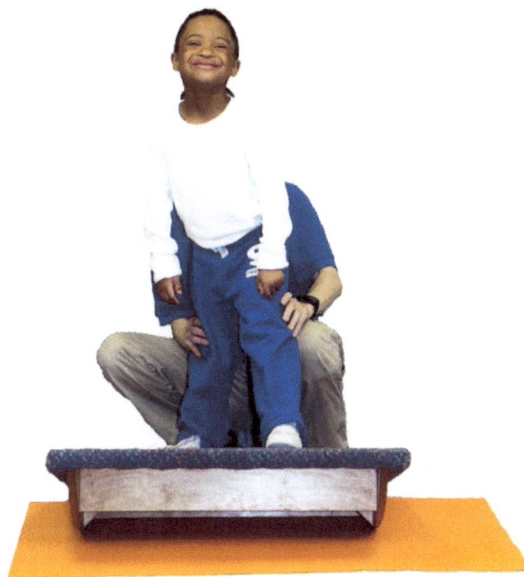

5. WEDGE STANDING

I love this activity. Determine what degree wedge your child can tolerate without falling off. This is a pre-manufactured wedge for dorsiflexed standing. The angle is pretty steep, so I often lessen the wedge's angle by placing a book or board under the heel end of the wedge. The thicker the book, the more it decreases the wedge's incline and makes it easier for the child to stand. Sometimes I will allow the child to stand on the wedge with their back to a wall, but I don't prefer the activity that way. It makes the exercise more passive and less active.

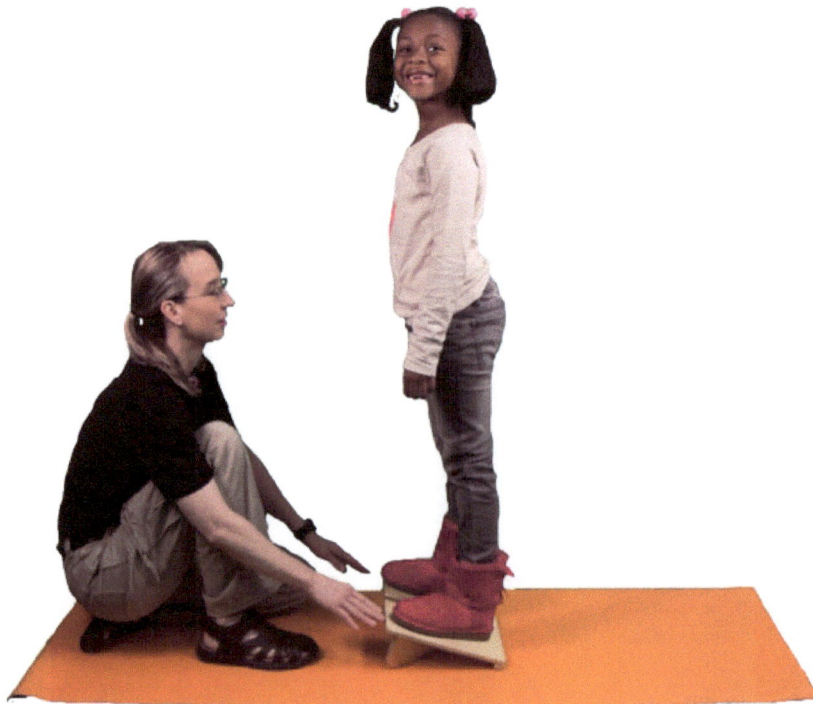

6. WEDGE STANDING AND PLAYING

If just standing is too easy, I like playing an activity while the child stands on the incline. I like remote-controlled car play, video gameplay, or hitting back and forth a tetherball or a balloon with a paddle. The more dynamic the game, the more active the dorsiflexors are.

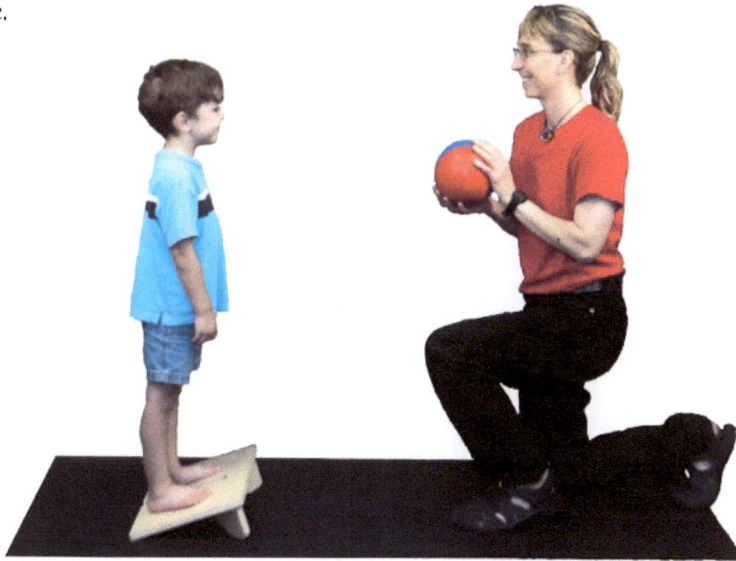

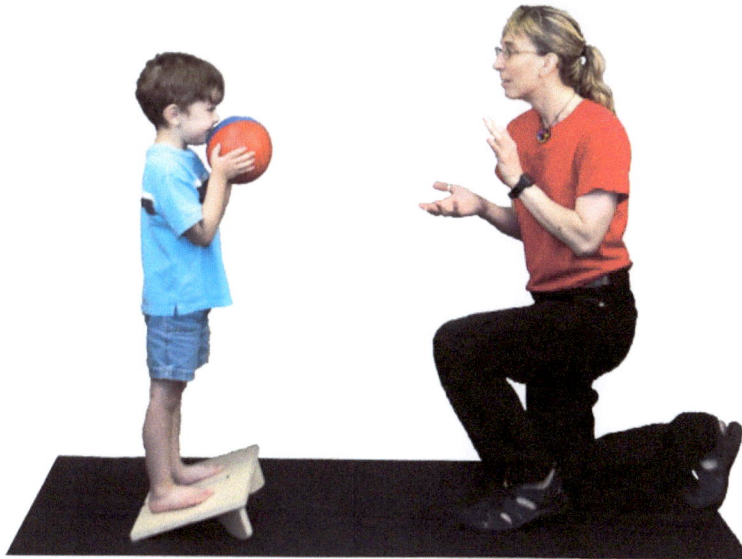

7. STANDING SCOOTER BOARD PUSH

Children are challenged to get dorsiflexion to clear their feet as they go forward. For my toe walkers, I emphasize heels down as they push. If this needs to be a little easier, I put a 4" bench on top of the scooter board. Assuming your scooter board is rectangular like ours at the clinic, make sure the bench's ends go to the front and back versus side to side. This arrangement makes it less likely for the bench to fall off the scooter board. For less-skilled children, I cinch down the bench with a belt firmly. I usually grab another scooter board and go with my clients. I have noticed that children often have trouble decelerating--so watch out for heels getting painfully charged.

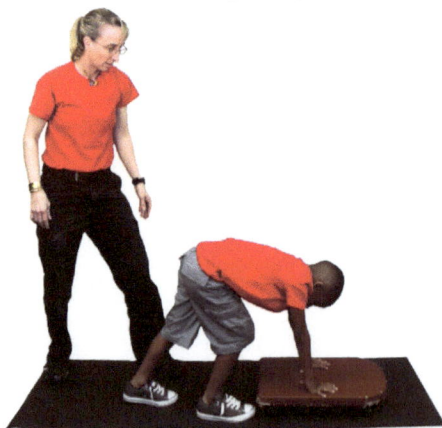

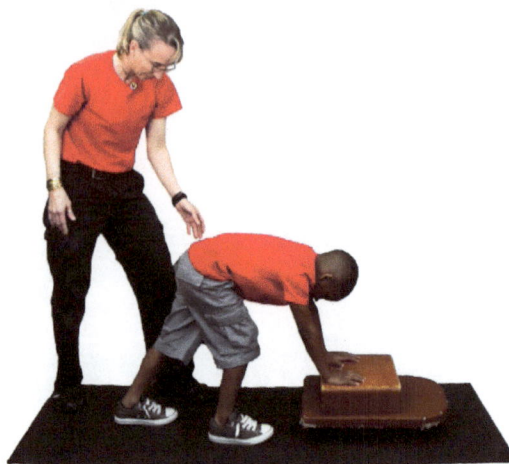

8. BEAR WALK, HEELS DOWN

This activity is harder than the previous one because the child's hands
are all the way down on the ground as opposed to a little higher on
a scooterboard. Of course, the floor is easier in some ways because
the floor is much more stable than the scooterboard. The child must
dorsiflex his feet to clear his feet to take each step. Again, I request my
toe walkers keep their heels down, which usually requires end range
dorsiflexion.

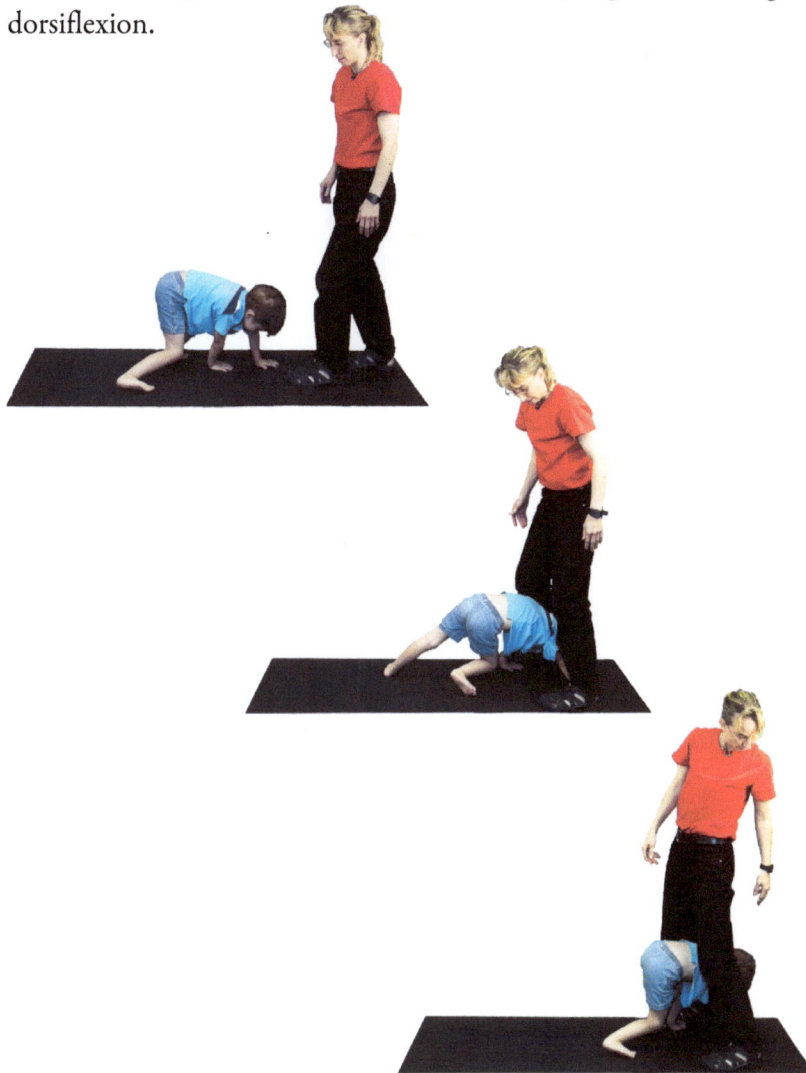

9. INCHWORM

For the inchworm, a child starts in the bear position and walks out just the hands until the child can't go any further. Then he walks his feet up as close as he can to his hands. In this photo sequence, I am helping my model get his heels down. The child must actively dorsiflex to be able to clear the foot for the next step.

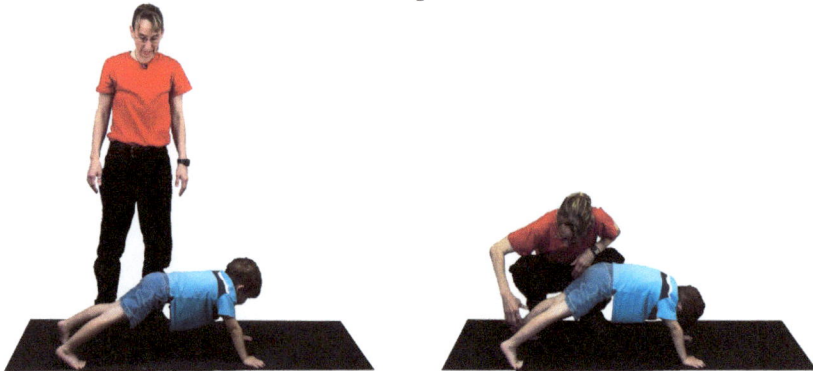

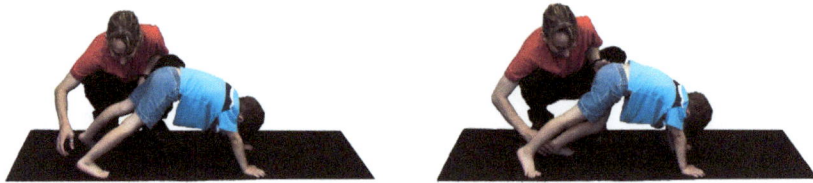

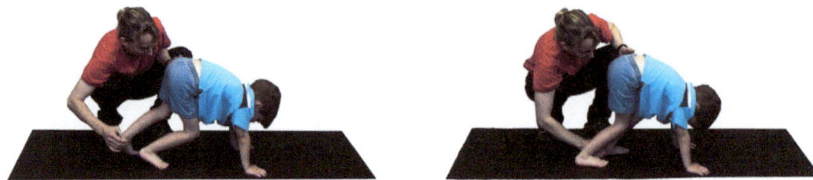

10. STEP WITH EXAGGERATED HEEL STRIKE

I simply have the child step, emphasizing toe-up instead of foot flat at floor contact/heel strike. Some children require a walker, hands held, or parallel bars for success. Others are strong enough to perform this without assistance. Here I have a squeak toy to hit with her heel. I have also used a keyboard.

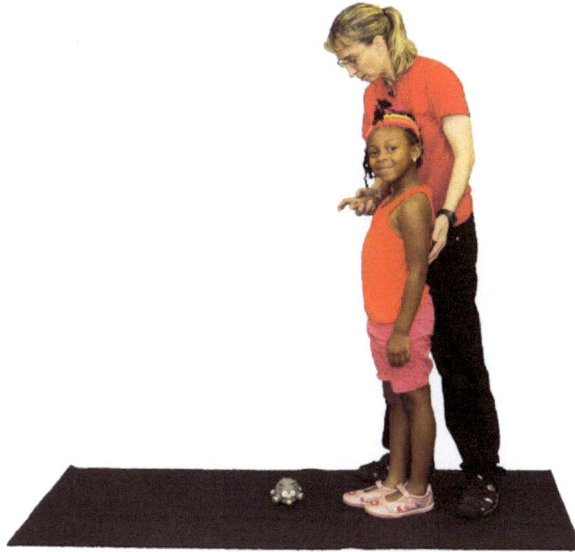

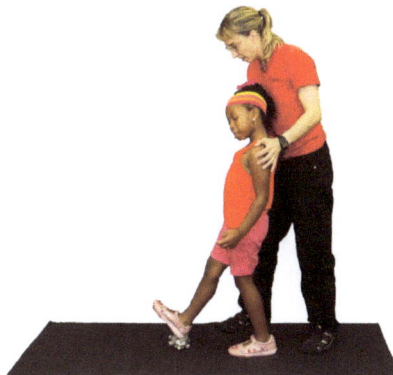

11. CHOOSE A TOY WITH HEEL, STANDING

In this activity, I place a toy with pieces on the floor in front of my client. I do this most often with those shape oreo cookies--but any toy with parts like stacking cups, a ring stander, or puzzles will work. The child stays in one place and must select which piece she wants next by touching it only with her heel. For success, a child may need upper extremity support, such as a hand held, upright poles, or a wall beside her.

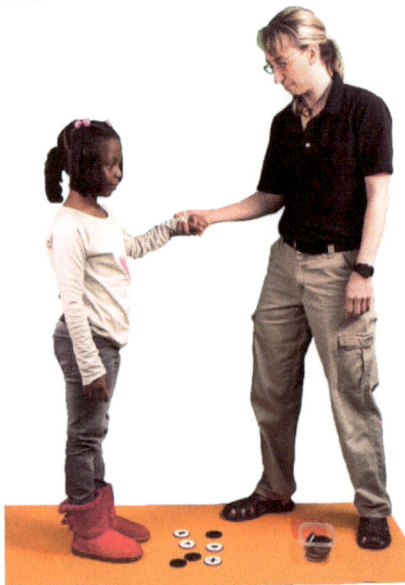

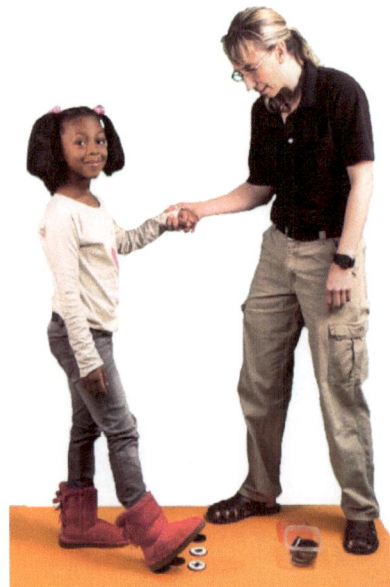

12. WRITE WITH YOUR FOOT

For children who know their alphabet, this is a good activity. I have a
whole set of alphabet letters. We go through each one, letter by letter.
The child can do the letter in the air, but sometimes I have to hold the
letter up in front of her toes for the child to trace. You can also play a
game in which the child writes a word one letter at a time. You have
to try to figure out what the word is by the movement of her foot.
Sometimes this works best if I limit the options to words that I have
written on the dry erase board. Or the child must keep it in a category
(like animals) to help me out a little.

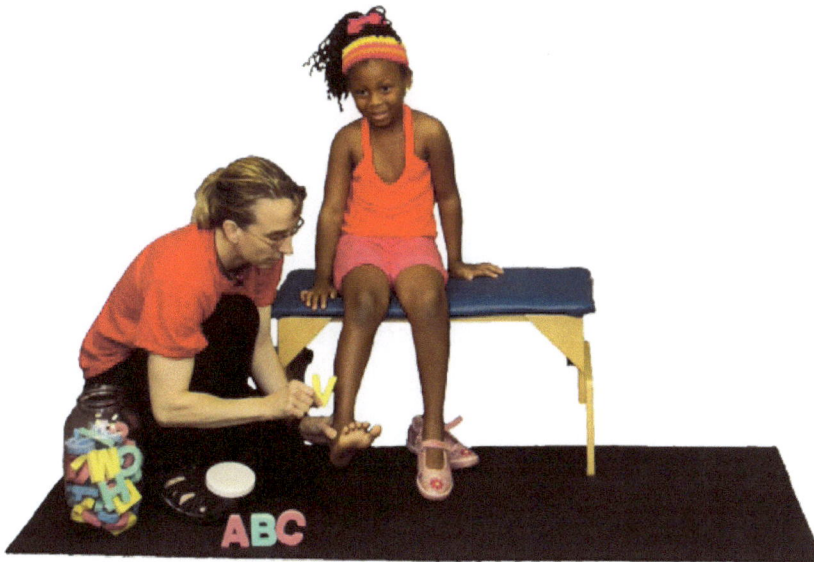

13. SEATED DORSIFLEXION, KNEE FLEXED

Dorsiflexion tends to be a little easier sitting than standing. The child sits on a bench. Here, I had my model start with a fairly extended leg and had him dorsiflex. I usually do ten repetitions and then have the child flex his knee a little bit more. More knee flexion effectively changes the start position to slightly more dorsiflexed, making the exercise a little more challenging. I have the child perform ten more repetitions, flex his knee a little more, and repeat. I continue this until the child is no longer able to dorsiflex his foot.

Sometimes I do a 15-second speed test comparing one foot to the other. Kids like this kind of competition. Make sure the heel stays down on this exercise. I often have to hold it down to ensure there is no cheating by lifting the entire leg. You can measure the amount of knee flexion and the number of repetitions performed for documentation purposes.

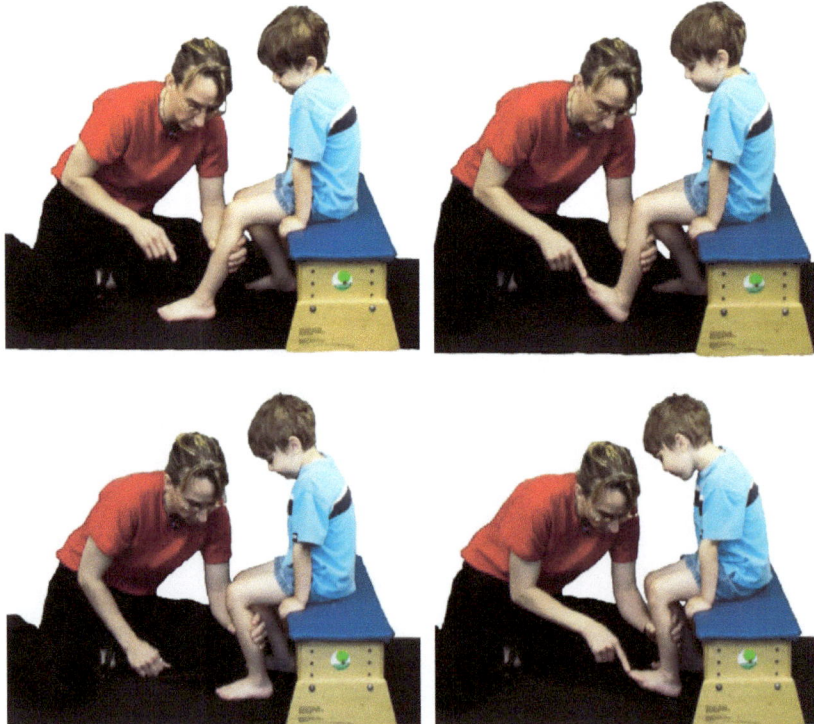

14. DORSIFLEXION LEANING ON A WALL

I have the child stand with his back to the wall with his feet away from the wall. I measure the distance from his heel to the wall for documentation purposes. When a child is successful with ten repetitions dorsiflexing his feet and clearing the forefoot from the floor, I ask the child to move the foot slightly closer to the wall. I measure the distance and repeat. I use a goniometer, ruler, or index card to swing underneath his forefoot to make sure it has completely cleared the floor. Often I will have a parent or sibling play along too. When the heels get close to the wall, this gets challenging. He may need to dorsiflex one foot at a time to be able to clear the forefoot from the floor. Make sure the child puts his foot down between each repetition. As the child starts to max out their active range of motion, I always hold the heels down. A common substitution is hiking the hip to clear the entire foot instead of dorsiflexing the foot. Or sometimes, clients extend/dorsiflex their toes instead of getting ankle movement. Pass the goniometer back far enough under the foot to ensure the entire forefoot clears the floor.

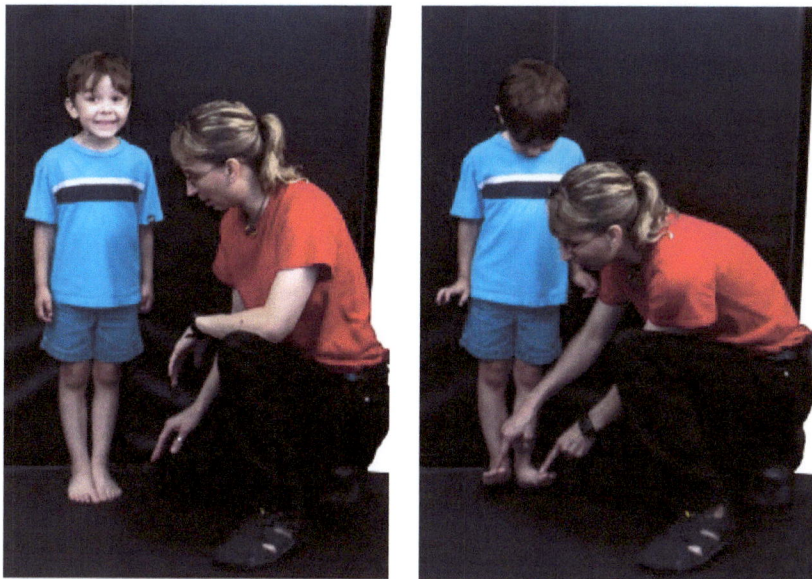

15. DECLINE TO INCLINE DORSIFLEXION

This exercise is similar to the previous one. But here, the child does not stand with her back to the wall. I start with the child standing on a decline. Here I made a decline by having the child stand with her heels on a book. The child dorsiflexes her feet 10x. Then I have her move to a lower decline (or a smaller book) and repeat. I usually have the child stand on a book that is ~1 inch (2.5 cm) thick, then ½ inch (1 cm) thick, then ¼ inch (0.5 cm) thick. My goal is for the child to stand flat on the floor and dorsiflex ten times. If the child needs more challenge, I put the same progressively thicker books now under her toes and have her dorsiflex her feet 10x. Without the wall behind them, my clients tend to cheat by flexing at the hip, which tilts their tibia posteriorly, making dorsiflexion easier. You see this classic cheat even with my neurotypical model by the last book height.

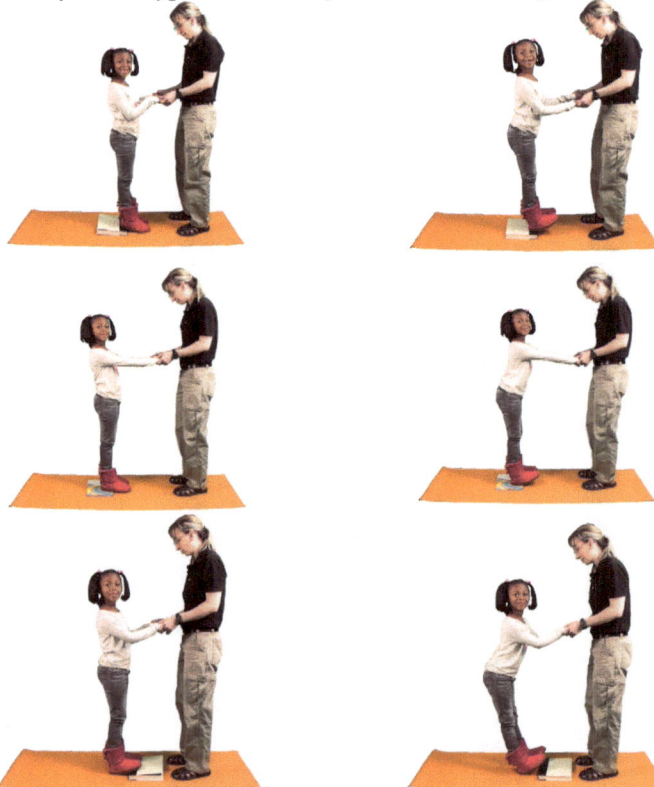

16. SHIN PULL UPS.

This exercise requires a motivated cooperative child. To start, a child leans back slightly against you or a wall or any other upright surface, emphasis on slightly. Keeping the body straight, the child pulls back up to upright standing using dorsiflexion. This is super hard. The lever arm of the body makes this exercise a powerful dorsiflexion strengthener. In another version, the child stands with her forefeet lodged under something. She leans back and comes back to upright. I do these at the gym with my toes under the exercise machines. Spot the child closely with this version. It is easy to go back too far and lose control.

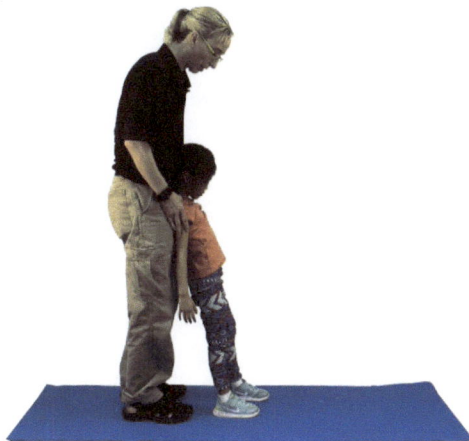

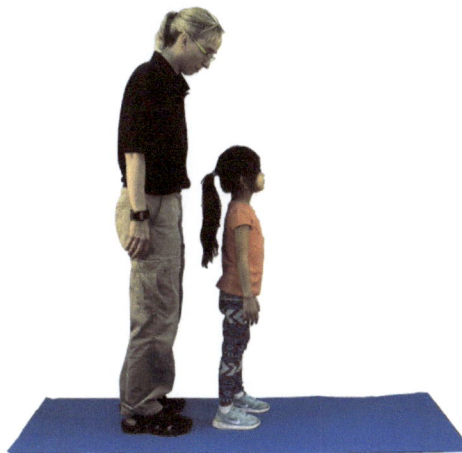

17. HEEL-TOE WALK

I work a great deal on a heel-toe gait pattern with my clients. I work on this pattern on the floor or the treadmill. Often I have to give more support than usual for my client to focus on the heel-toe gait pattern. When she is successful, I start withdrawing the extra help. For some of my clients, longer step lengths make the difference. My marginal walkers with cerebral palsy often need to focus on terminal knee extension instead of a steppage gait pattern for success. I start slow and work to increase speed or the number of correct steps with a heel-toe gait pattern. Sometimes the heel strikes only slightly before the rest of the foot. In this case, I may need to lay on the floor in front to observe (usually further out than is pictured). Or I have a parent in front to be the judge. To get the best view of the feet, I may sit or lie prone on a scooter board in front and push myself backward as the client walks toward me. I love the treadmill to practice this skill because it is easy to change the speed. I don't have to chase my client around to verify the gait pattern. I can also physically assist as needed, hand over foot.

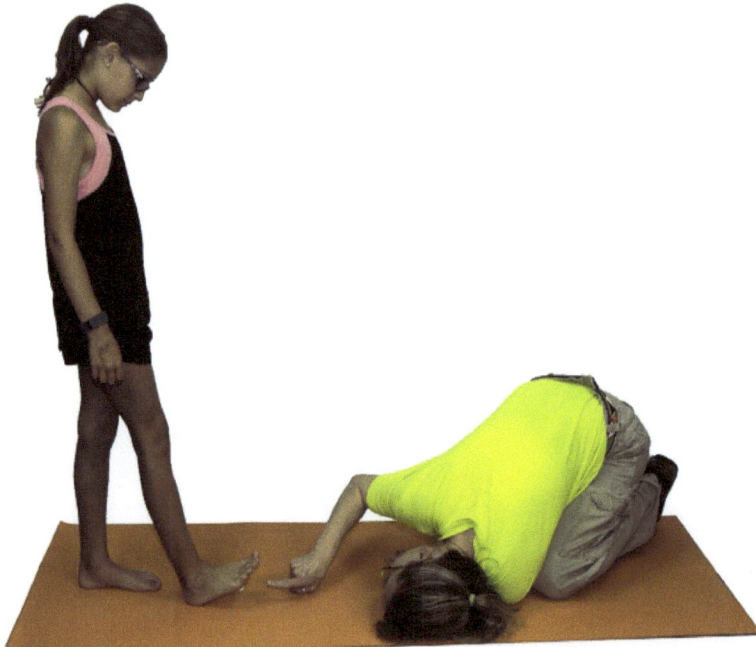

18. HEEL WALK

For successful heel walking, a child may need to hold a walker, have
one or two hands held, or have a hand on the wall. I do this exercise
two ways. I tape a squeaker to the bottom of a child's forefoot and
count the number of steps until I hear a squeak. Or I lay on the
floor and watch to see how many heel walk steps the child performs
correctly. The number of steps I determine visually is always the
subject of some debate, including some "No, I didn't touch down!"
and "Yes, you did." The auditory cue of the squeaker is much less
debatable. I record how many steps, how far, or how long the child can
heel walk without error. I like to perform this exercise with the child.
Ugh. My dorsiflexors get tired well before many of my toe walkers do.

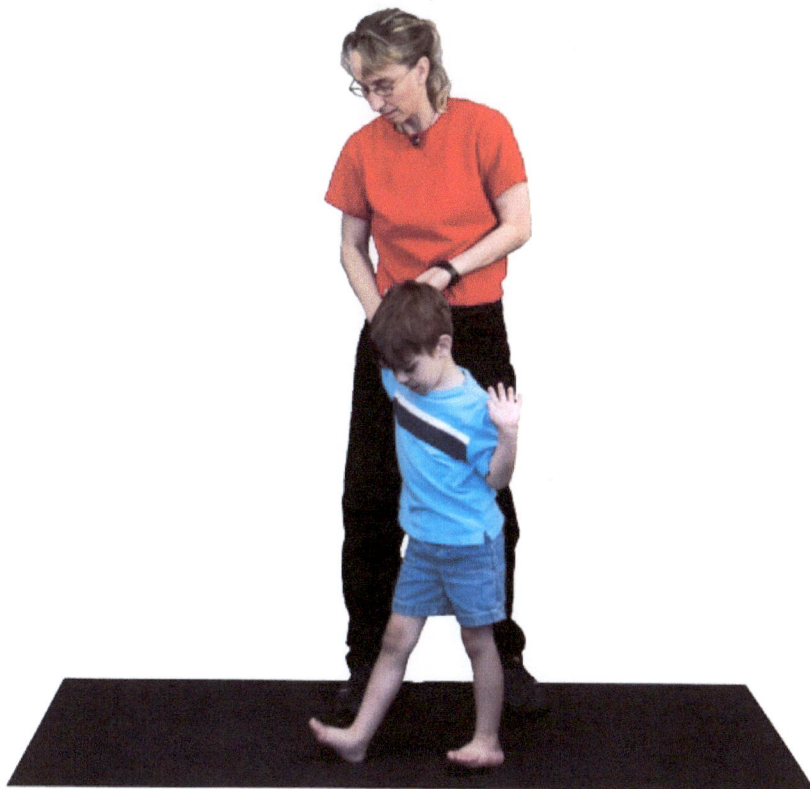

19. DORSIFLEXION TO ROLL THE CARS

Some kids love cars. If you can include a car, then the activity will be a success. This model was that way. I put a board on his forefeet as he sat. With the car placed at the top of the board, when he dorsiflexed his feet, he lifted the board, and down the car went. The heavier the board, the harder this activity is. This board is pretty heavy, but it didn't take much of a lift to get the car to go. He was happy anyway. More knee flexion also makes this activity harder.

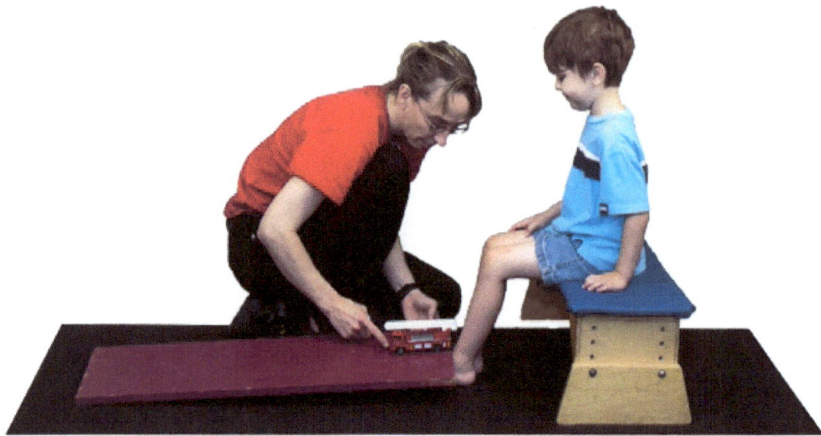

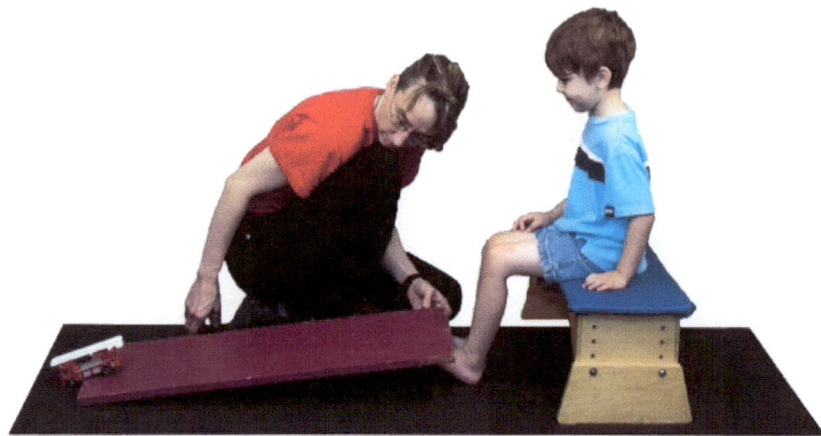

20. HEEL WALK FROM A ROLLING CHAIR

Dorsiflexion with knee flexion is much easier than dorsiflexion
with knee extension. In this exercise, I ask the child to propel herself
forward while seated on a rolling chair, pulling only with her heels.
The toes should be up. This activity is more manageable on a
smooth floor and much harder on carpeting. The hamstrings are the
workhorse of this exercise, but the anterior tibialis is working hard too.

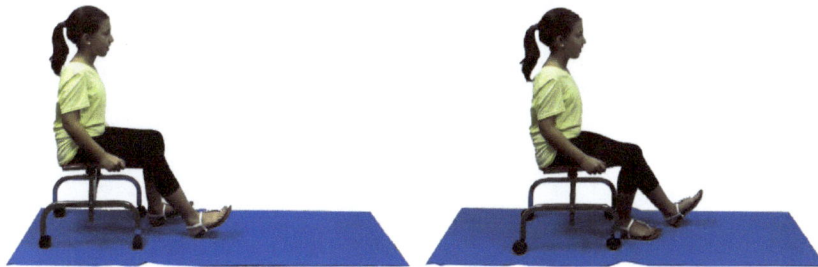

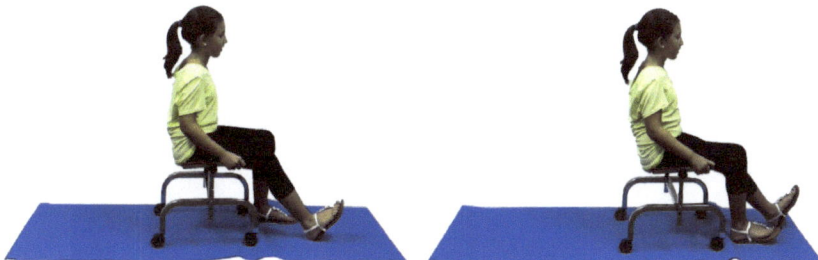

21. SEATED HEEL PRESS

If you press down with your toes in sitting, you are using your plantarflexors. If you press down on your heels, your dorsiflexors are working. I manually resist the heels going down.

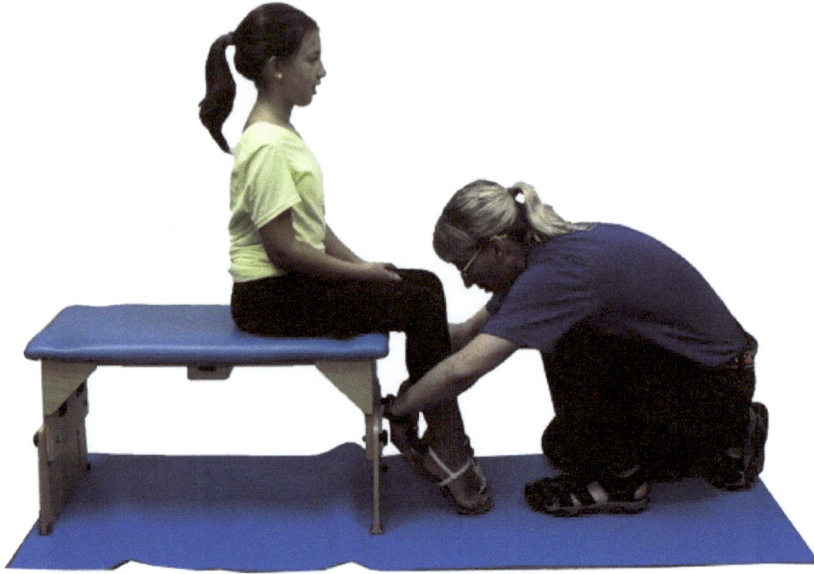

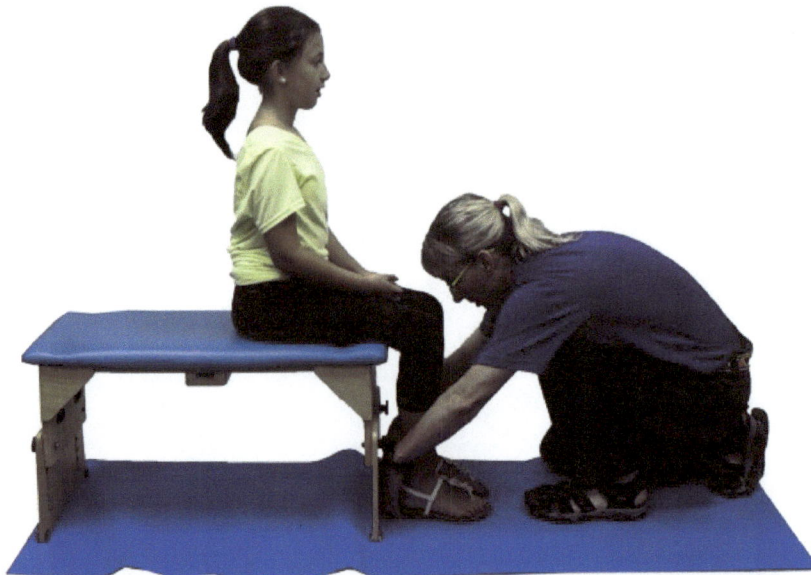

22. WEDGE STAND ON ONE FOOT

Usually, I let the child get accustomed to the wedge on both feet
before lifting one leg. The slope of the wedge makes this activity
harder or easier. If needed, I put a book under the wedge on the
heel side to make it not as steep. I usually simply count to 10 or 30.
But I have had a rare client that can do this and hit back and forth a
tetherball or a balloon with me.

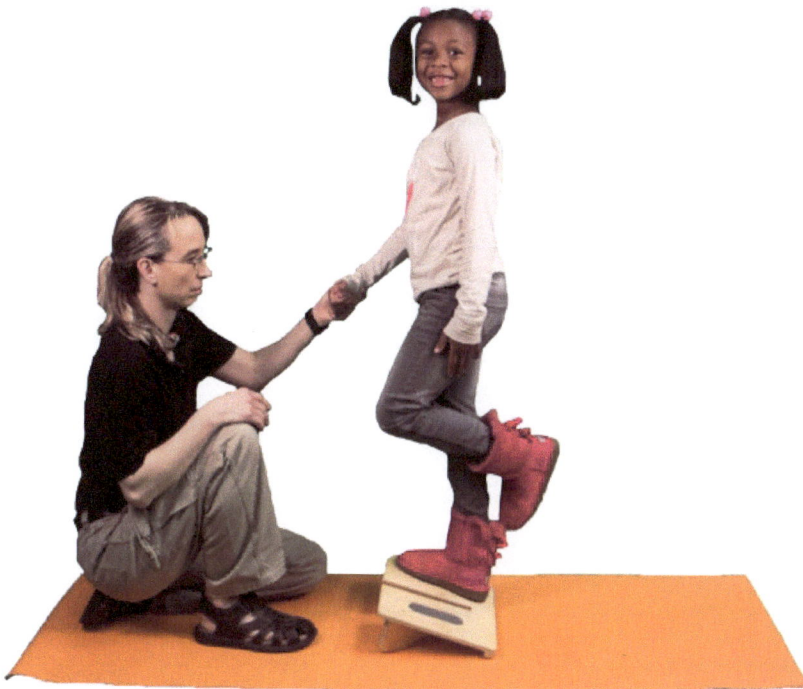

23. HOLDING SQUATTING

My model here can hold squatting without much effort, but many of my clients are unable. For some people, simply holding a squat requires the dorsiflexors to fire strongly to keep them from falling posteriorly. Cheats include having the feet turned out, having the knees out very wide (to turn out the feet), and reaching way forward with the arms to counterbalance and hold the position. You can decide which of these cheats you allow or don't. If a child can hold the squat for 10-30 seconds with heels on a 1" (2.5 cm) thick book, I progress to the ½" (1 cm) thick book, then the ¼" (0.5 cm) thick book, then the floor. I emphasize that the heels must be down.

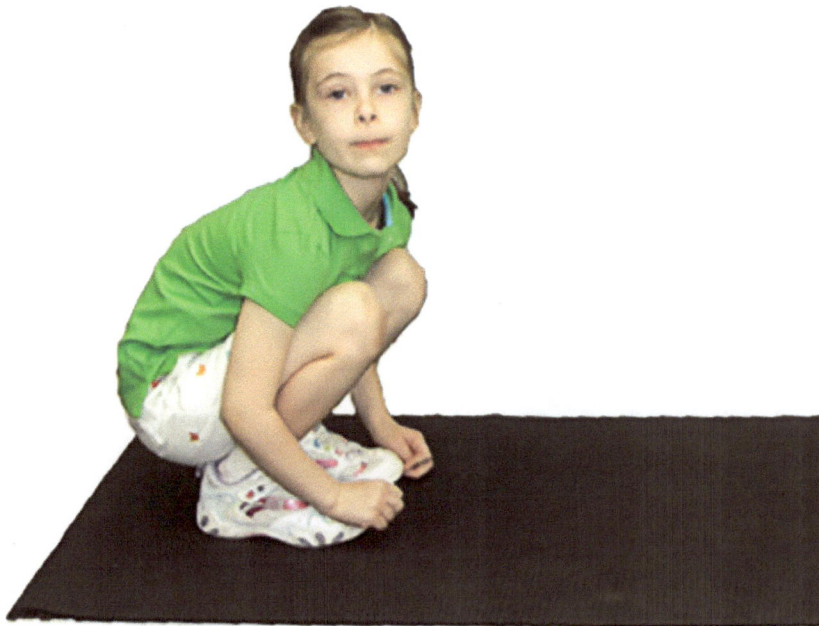

24. SQUAT WALK

Dorsiflexing the foot at end range to step while squat walking is challenging, especially for diplegic children and toe walkers. I can make this a little easier by holding one or two hands. I typically only have the children squat walk 6-15'. (2-5 m) Again, I emphasize that the heels must go down flat with the squat walk.

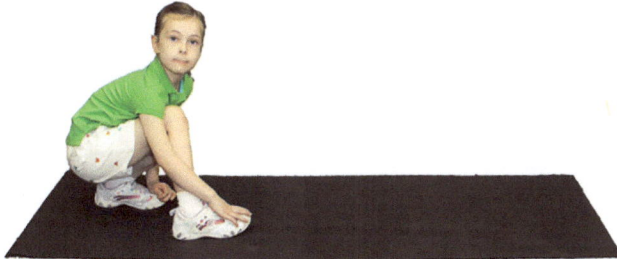

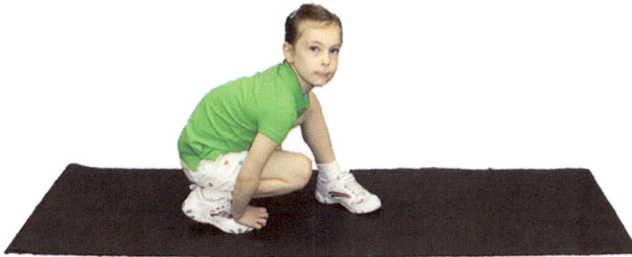

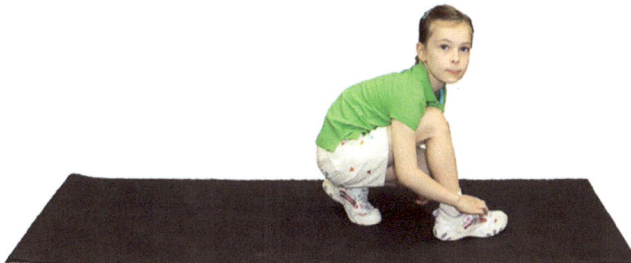

III. INVERSION

THE ANKLE INVERTERS PULL THE bottom of the foot in toward the middle. Activating your inverters makes you stand on the outside of your foot. Strong and balanced inverters and everters are critical for moving on uneven surfaces, lateral movement, and balance. Weakness in the inverters make individuals more at risk for ankle injuries. As pediatric physical therapists, we often deal with weakness in the inverters associated with cerebral palsy or toe walking. This chapter includes a wide variety of exercises to improve ankle inversion strength and control.

* * *

1. SUPINE INVERSION, MANUALLY RESISTED

The only downside to this exercise is my client cannot see the movement from flat supine. So, sometimes I prop the child up on a pillow or allow the child to sit up, leaning back on his arms to watch the movement. Or if I think the child has good body awareness, I may simply take his foot through the motion and say, "It feels like this..." for a couple of repetitions. If a child can get any inversion, it is usually from the extreme everted position back toward midline. Often I can resist from the everted position to neutral and then have to assist from neutral to the inverted position. In any case, I give as much resistance as a child can take and as little assistance as possible. Sometimes I make a competition. I tell the child he has 10 seconds to get to the "feet in" position. I make a good show of resisting and usually lose. I don't let the child win every time, or the fun is gone.

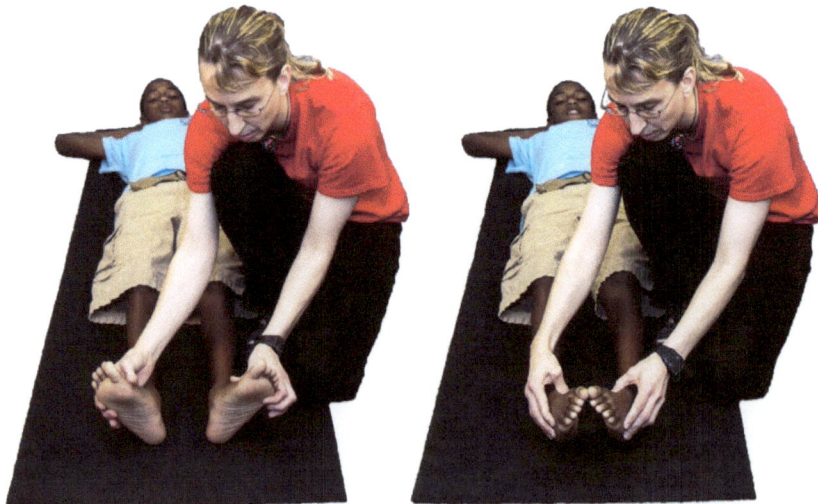

2. WRITE THE ALPHABET WITH YOUR FEET

For children who know their alphabet, this is a good activity. Only the letter, "I", is straight up and down, so all the other letters will get some inversion.

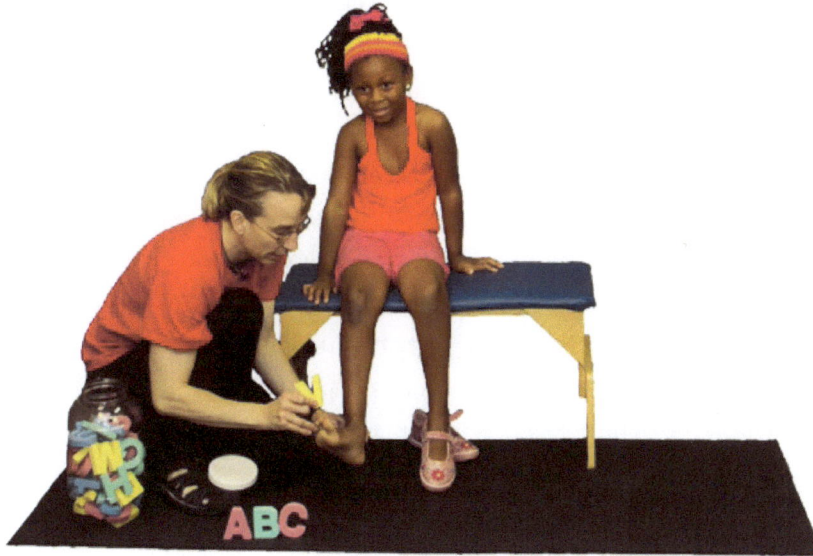

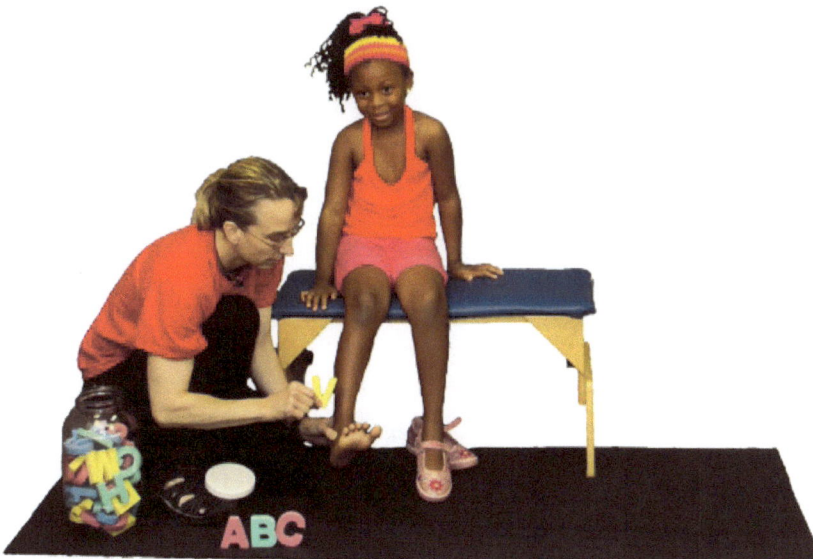

3. SEATED INVERSION, MANUALLY RESISTED

I use one hand to provide resistance/assistance to the foot. The thumb on the other hand is the target. I start the child in extreme eversion and cue them to bring their foot into inversion. I position the target hand with my pinky on the shin. The child inverts to touch my thumb. This ensures that wherever the shin goes, my target goes too. Children often try to bring their leg medially in their inversion attempts. I check a child's range first to find a realistic target position. Some children, particularly those with cerebral palsy, have no idea how to move their foot into inversion. I may have to help them move their foot through the entire range. I find plantarflexion control develops first, then dorsiflexion, then eversion/inversion. I perform this activity concentrically and eccentrically. The child inverts his foot to end range. The child resists for a ten count as I pull it into eversion toward a target on the opposite side. Sometimes I use electric stimulation to help a child get the feeling of this movement.

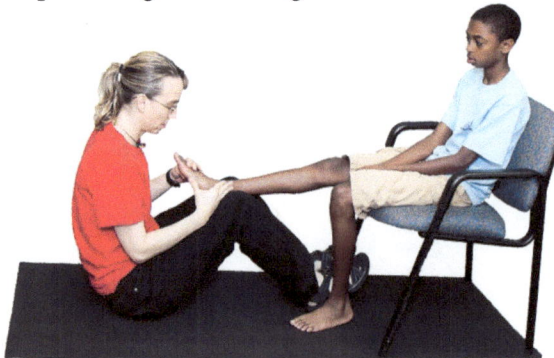

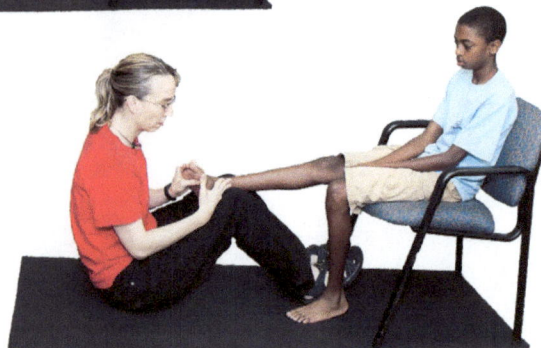

4. ELASTIC BAND, RESISTED INVERSION

I typically use manual resistance, but sometimes I pull out the elastic band, especially if I think the child (with parent's assistance) might do this exercise at home. Sometimes, kids like the challenge of progressing up from the easiest color of theraband to the hardest. Here I am holding the elastic band, but I could also tie it off.

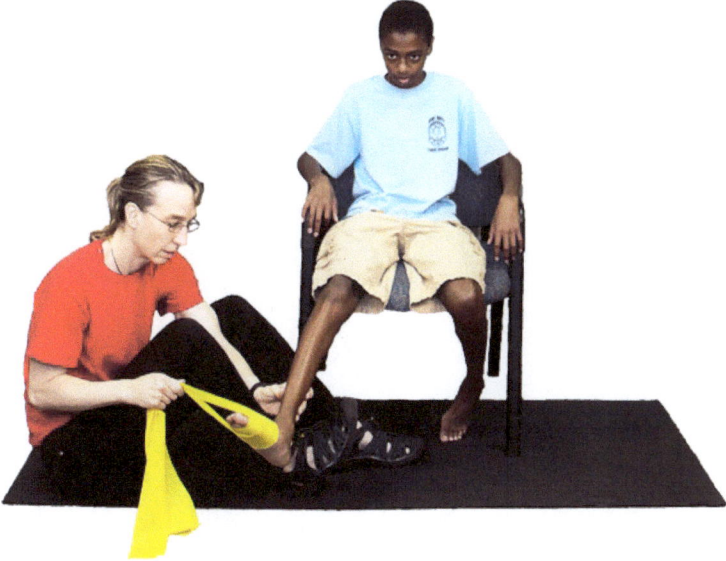

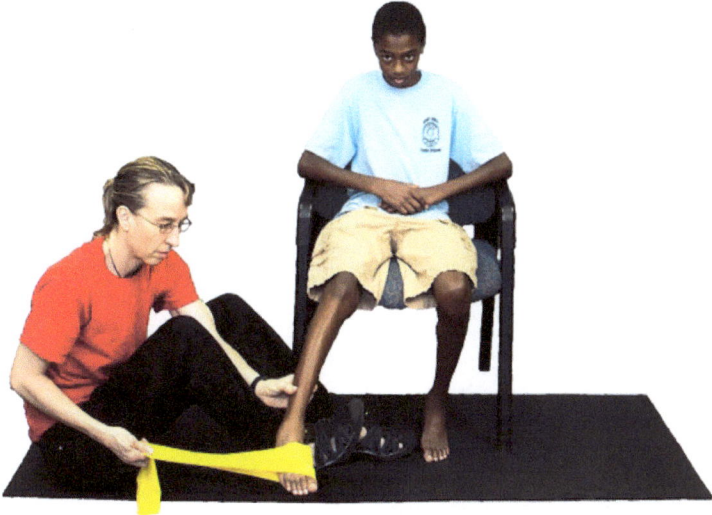

5. SEATED HEEL DOWN INVERSION

By having my client stabilize his foot on the floor, I get less cheating with hip adduction and internal rotation. Place the target carefully. I passively take the foot to the end range position to see how much movement is possible to help guide me in target placement. Alternately, you can start with the target very close to the foot and then work progressively up and farther in for more robust inversion.

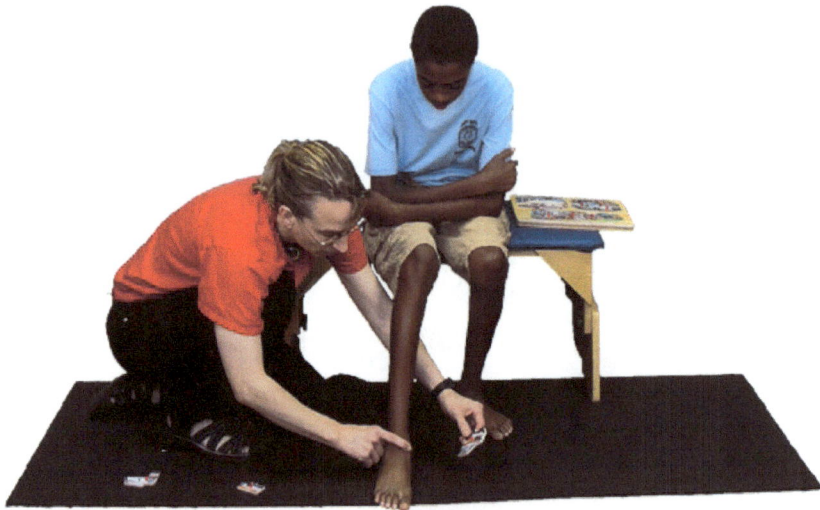

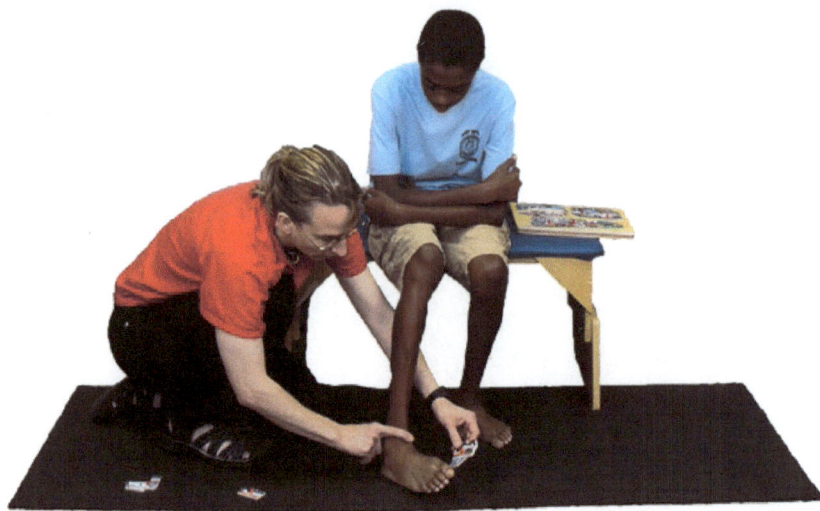

6. SEATED BALL PICK UP

Ok, I know, I know. This exercise gets hip flexion, hip adduction, hip external rotation--but also potentially some inversion, especially with an older cooperative kid who understands what you want. This exercise is too easy to cheat on if you think your client cannot understand, isolate the movement, and cooperate.

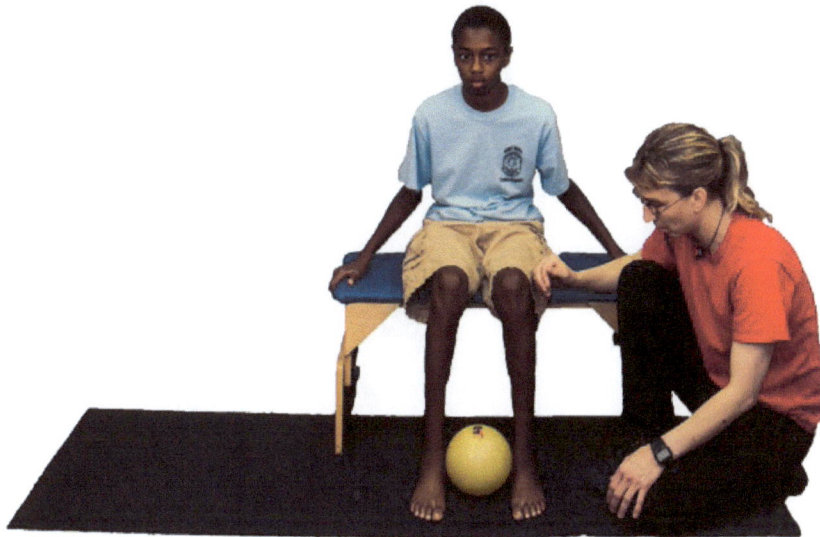

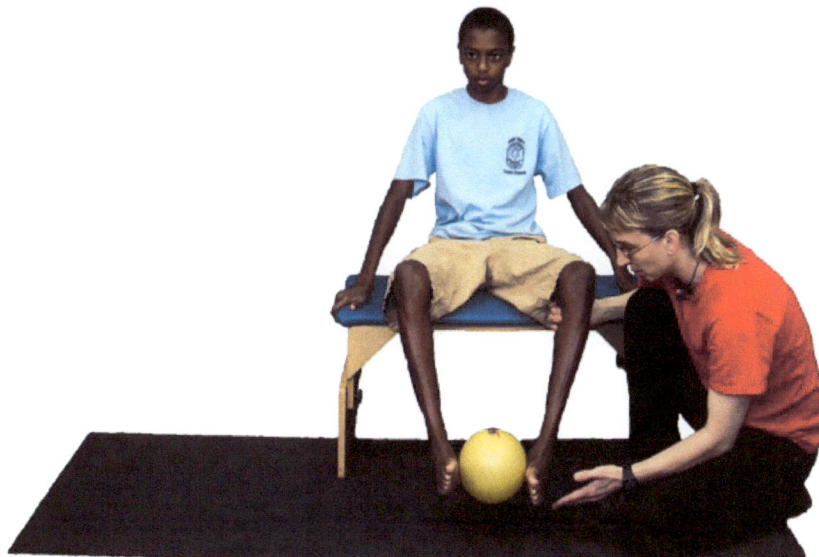

7. STANDING ON A SIDE SLANT

Due to the level of challenge, sometimes I have to start with two hands held, then progress to one hand held, and then have the client stand independently. Usually, the foot on the down side is working the hardest, strongly inverting. Decrease the difficulty by putting a book under the wedge on the lower side to decrease the slope. I time how long the child can stand and the angle of the wedge for documentation purposes.

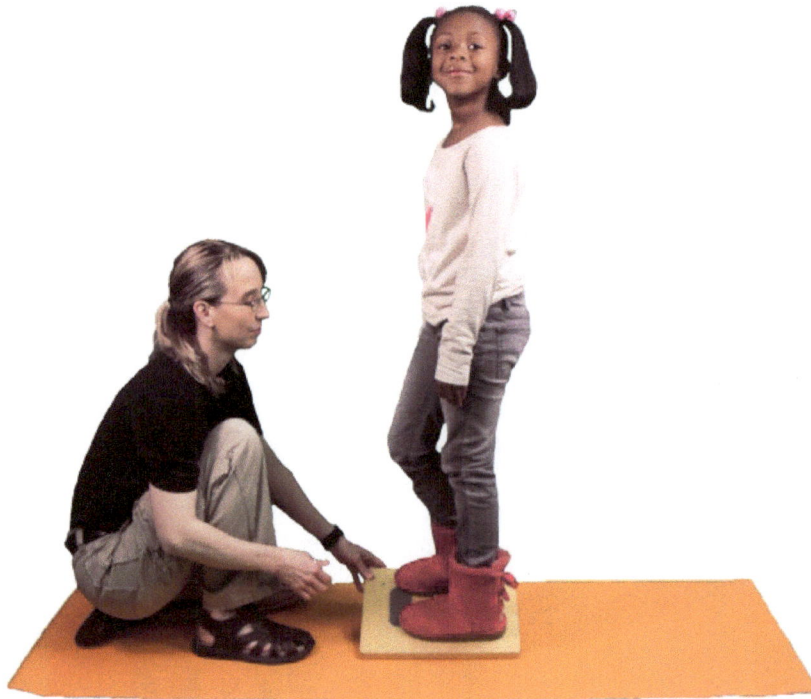

8. ONE FOOT STAND ON A SIDE SLANT

This can be a super challenging exercise. When you stand on one foot, you have more than doubled the work the foot is doing. To get inversion work, the child must stand on the foot closer to the bottom of the wedge as he stands sideways.

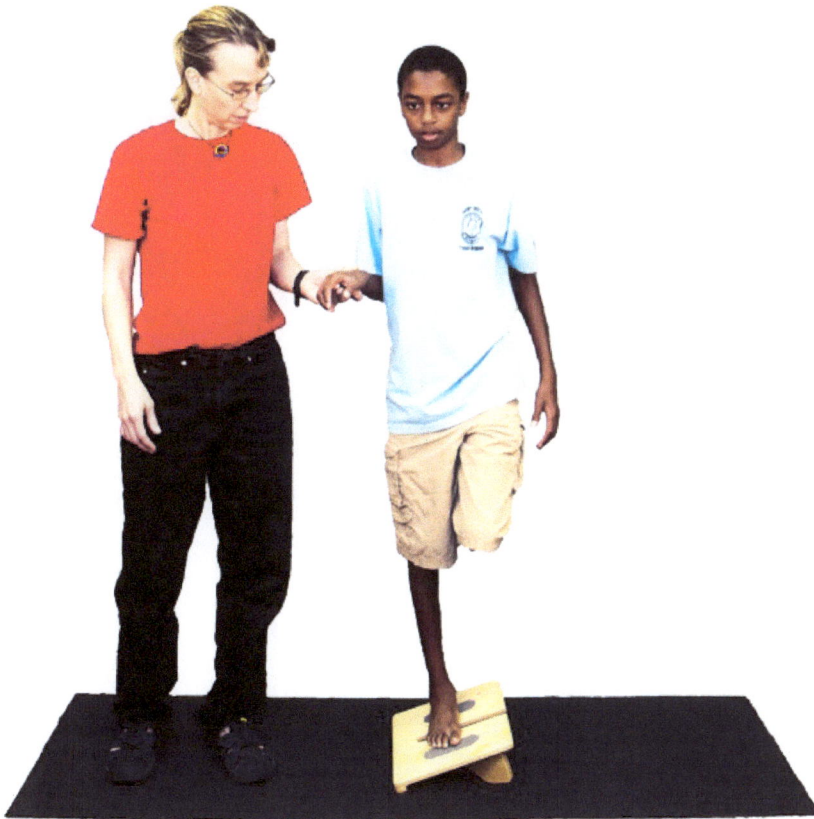

9. ACTIVE INVERSION STANDING

This activity requires strength, range, and balance. If this exercise is challenging, I let him hold onto something. Then I manually assist in inverting their feet. Sometimes I have to retreat to sitting. Often the movement is easier sitting without the weight bearing through the feet. I may also have the client perform one foot at a time instead of bilaterally. If the client has a better foot, I let him do that foot before the "tricky" foot.

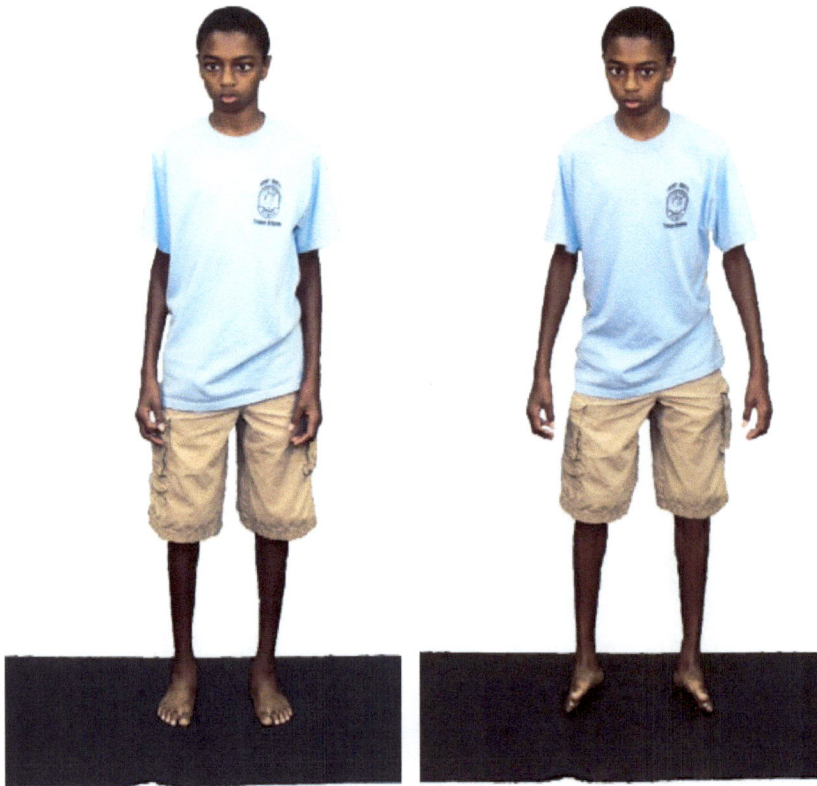

10. TOUCH BOTTOM OF THE FOOT

This activity requires a client who understands the movement and is cooperative. Because much of this movement is hip external rotation, choose this exercise with a client who understands how to emphasize inversion as well. I want my client to try to get the bottom of his foot facing up toward the ceiling.

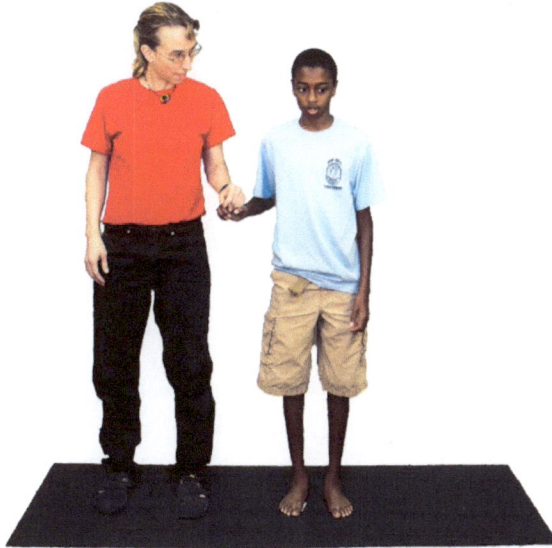

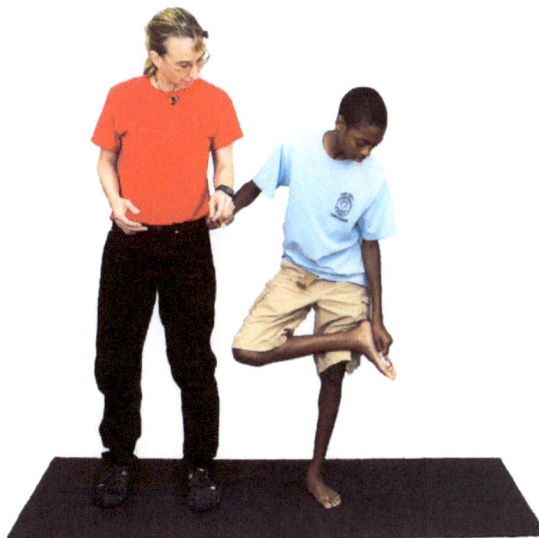

11. STANDING BOLSTER ROLL

This exercise requires some standing balance, unless of course you hold a hand or two. The right size bolster roll is essential. If the bolster is too small, it is hard to roll. If it is too large, my clients have trouble getting their foot on top. The client rolls the bolster side to side. It is very easy to cheat with this exercise and only get hip internal and external rotation. So this exercise requires a very cooperative client who understands the concepts of foot inversion and eversion and can concentrate on the movement.

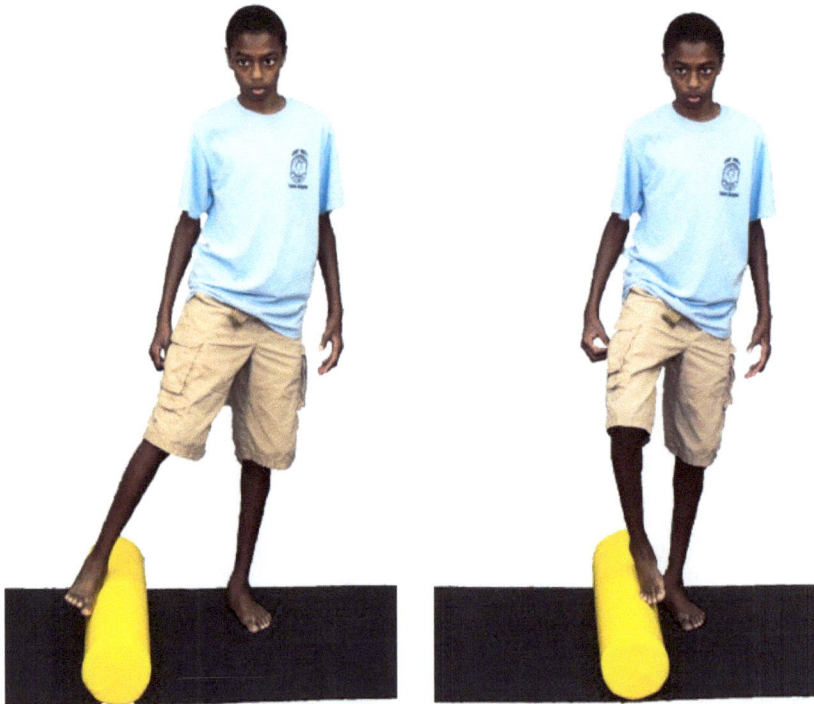

12. SIDE TO SIDE ON THE ROCKER BOARD

This activity gets several muscle groups--but it also includes inversion on the lower/more downhill foot. The higher/uphill foot gets eversion. One or two hands held may be necessary. I put the rocker board on the mat if I want slower and more controlled movements. I put the rocker board on a hard surface if I want quicker movements with less resistance. Narrower placement of the feet encourages more foot work.

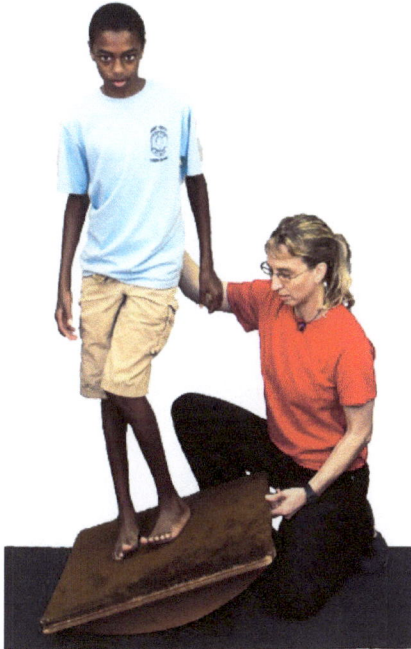

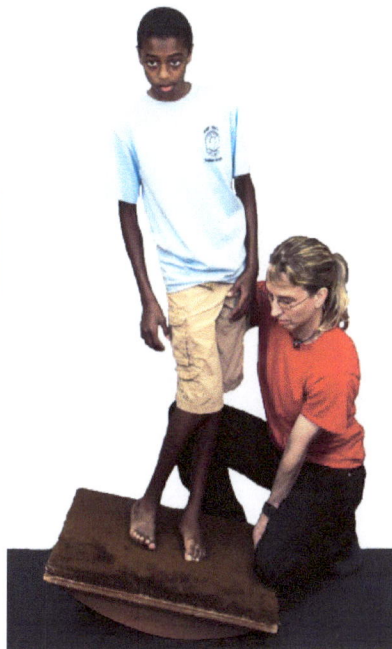

13. SIDE TO SIDE ROCK ON A BALANCE DISC

Again, multiple muscle groups are active, but these include inversion on the lower or downhill foot. The higher or more uphill foot gets eversion. The balance disc allows movement in all directions, making it harder for my children to control for strict inversion and eversion. But by the nature of the disc, the range of movement is limited. One or two hands held may be necessary.

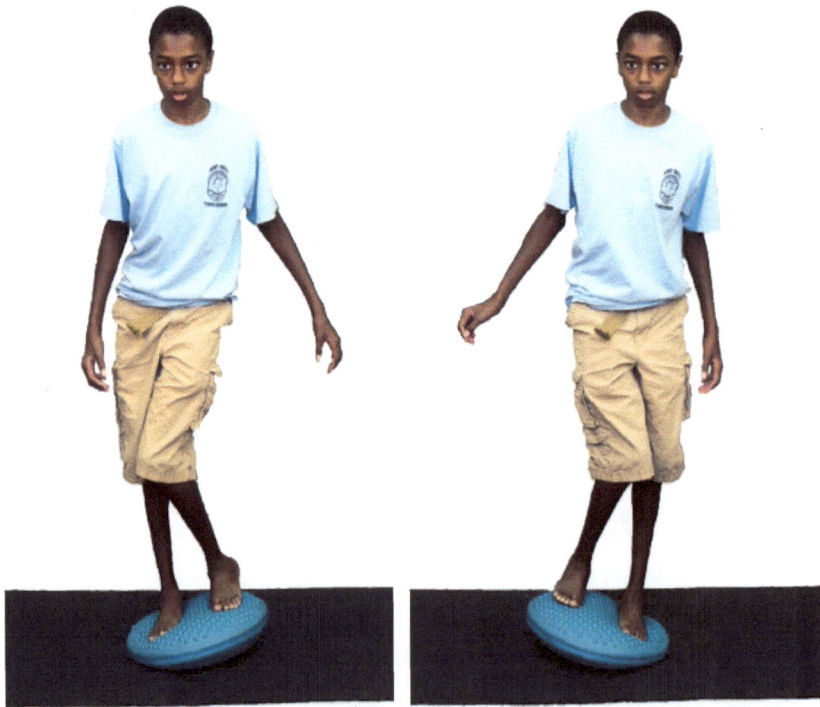

14. SIDE TO SIDE ROCK ON A POGO BALL

A pogo ball allows movement in all directions and thus is more challenging for my children to control for strict inversion and eversion. By the nature of the pogo/ball, the range of movement available is extreme and much harder for my clients to control. Again, one or two hands held may be necessary.

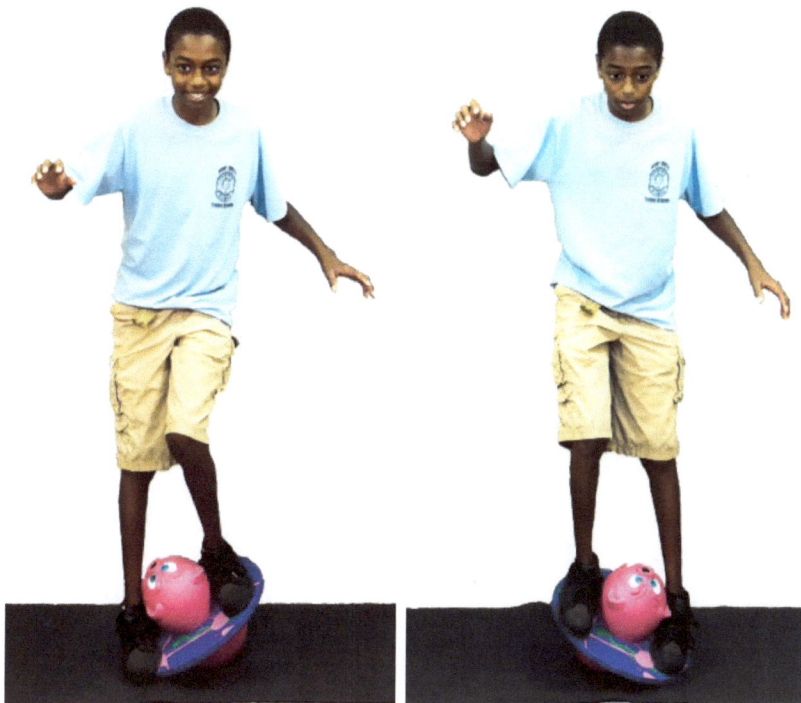

15. SIDEWAYS WIBBLE WOBBLE

In this exercise, the client moves sideways going on his toes, pivoting to the side, then going on his heels, and pivoting to the side again. I have the child go a distance to the right and then return to the left. This can be performed on one or two feet. If on one foot, then I let him put two hands on the wall to go sideways. For less challenge, the child wears socks, moves on a smooth floor, and holds a counter or tabletop. For the highest challenge, the kid wears tennis shoes and moves on carpeting without arm support.

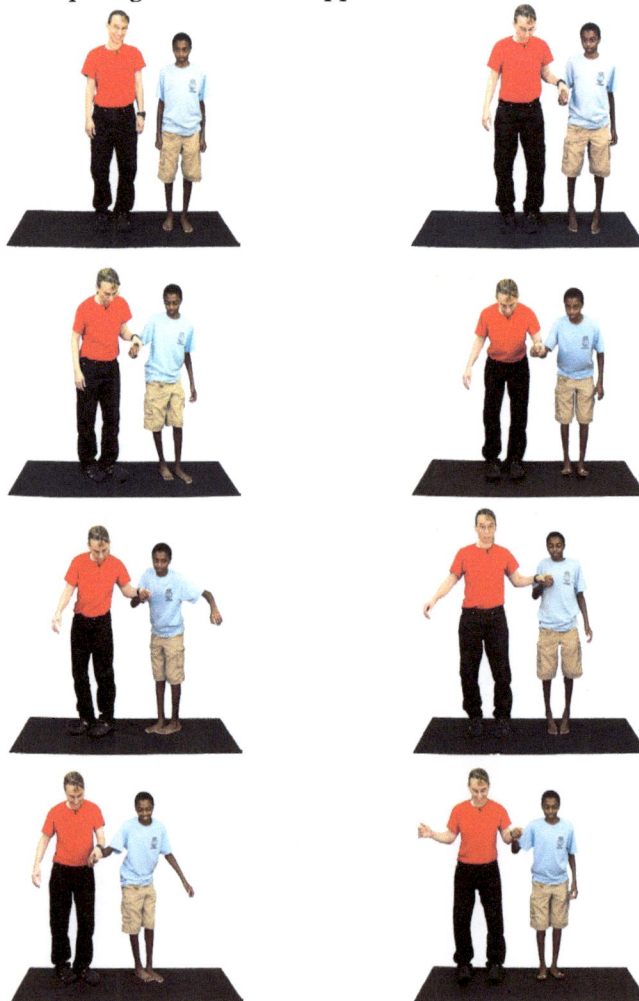

16. IN-LINE STRIDE STANDING

A narrow base of support encourages adduction/abduction and inversion/eversion balance reactions. To get the purest inversion/eversion make sure the feet are pointing straight ahead. Standing on a line helps the foot alignment.

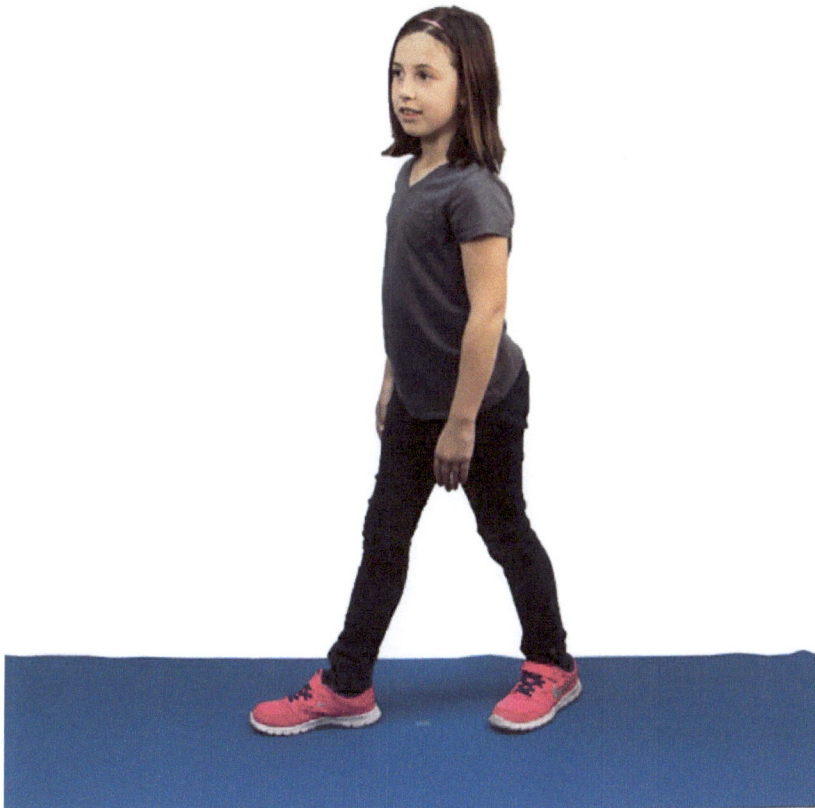

17. STANDING ON ONE FOOT

Standing on one foot is a wonderful way to work on inversion and eversion strength. Balance reactions are a full-body interaction, but the inverters and everters work powerfully to manage balance. Balance exercises deserve a whole book unto itself. Maybe I'll get to that in the future.

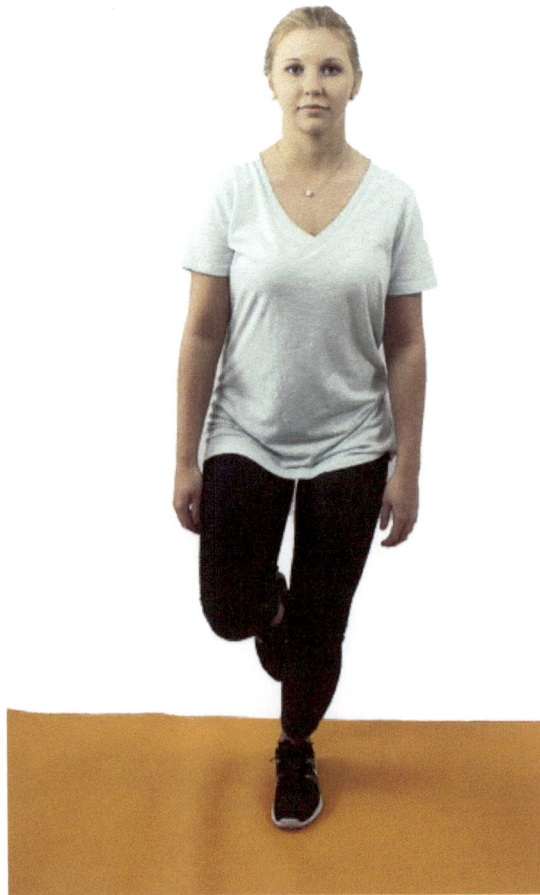

18. MEDIAL LATERAL MOVEMENTS IN SINGLE LEG STANCE

To encourage inversion and eversion in single leg stance, movements of the free leg in the sagittal plane encourage side to side balance reactions at the ankle which in turn encourage inversion and eversion muscle contractions.

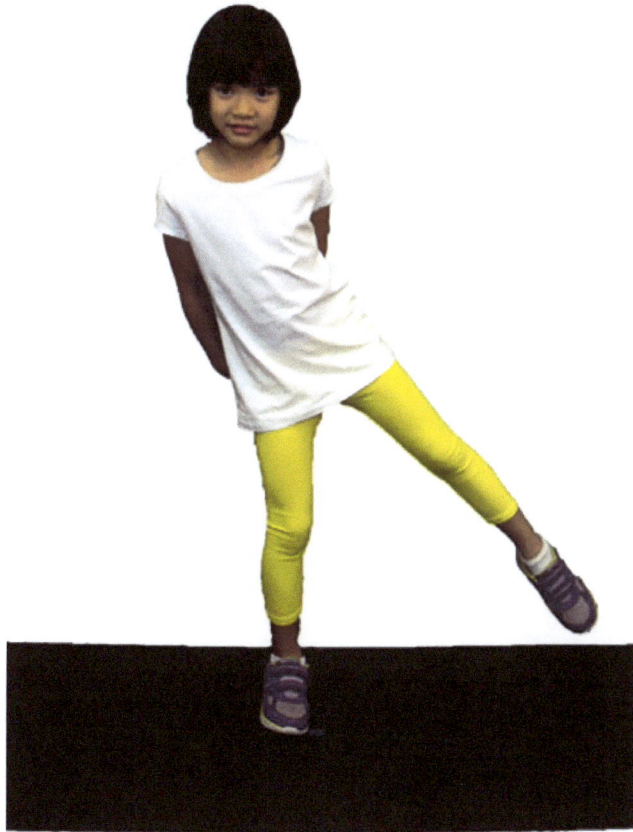

IV. EVERSION

THE ANKLE EVERTERS PULL THE bottom of the foot outward or away from the middle of your body. Activating your everters makes you stand more on the inside of your foot. Strong and balanced inverters and everters are critical for moving on uneven surfaces, lateral movement, and balance. Weakness in the everters make individuals more at risk for ankle sprains. As pediatric physical therapists, we often deal with weakness in the everters associated with cerebral palsy or toe walking. This chapter includes a wide variety of exercises to improve ankle eversion strength and control.

* * *

1. SUPINE EVERSION, MANUALLY RESISTED

Usually, I position myself sitting below my client's feet. I sit facing the child on the floor with my legs in a relatively wider ring position so that when the child everts his feet, he touches my feet conveniently there as a target. Here, I moved to the side to allow the exercise to be photographed more easily. Sometimes I prop the child upon a pillow or have him sit up to see the movement better. Or if I think the child has good body awareness, I may take his foot through the motion and say, "It feels like this..." for a couple of repetitions. If a child can get any eversion, it is usually from the extreme inverted position back toward midline. Often I resist from the inverted position to neutral and then assist from neutral to the everted position. Watch for substitution with hip external rotators.

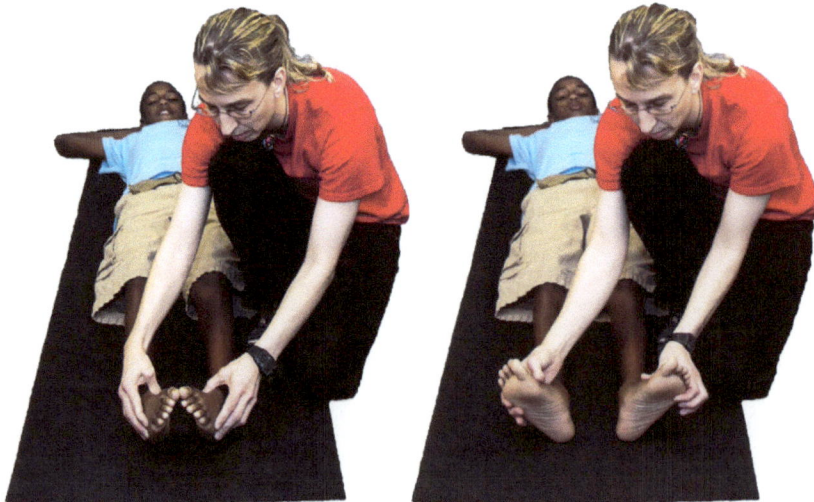

2. WRITE THE ALPHABET WITH YOUR FEET

Personally, I perform this exercise on an airplane on a long flight
to keep away the stiffness, swelling, and blood clots. What's good
for inversion is often good for eversion. To add some variety to this
exercise, you could have your client write the letter with her toe
pressing into rolled out playdo. Or she could press a coin with her big
toe on smooth flooring and write the letters.

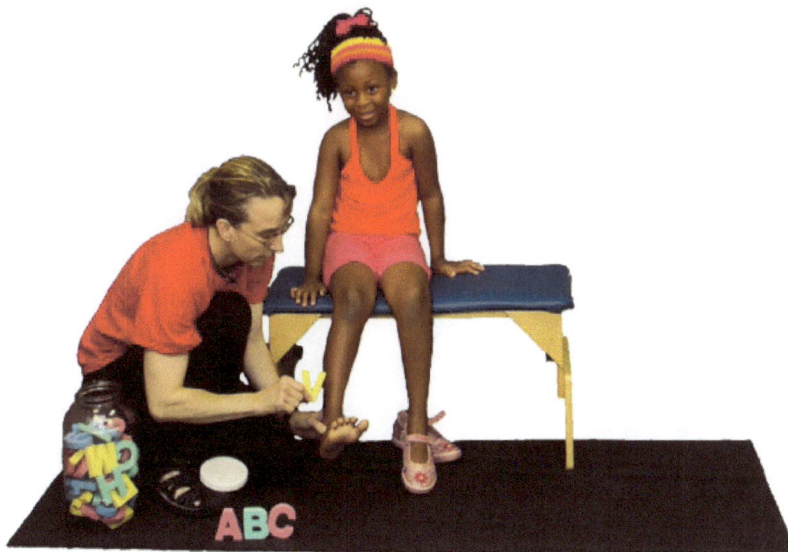

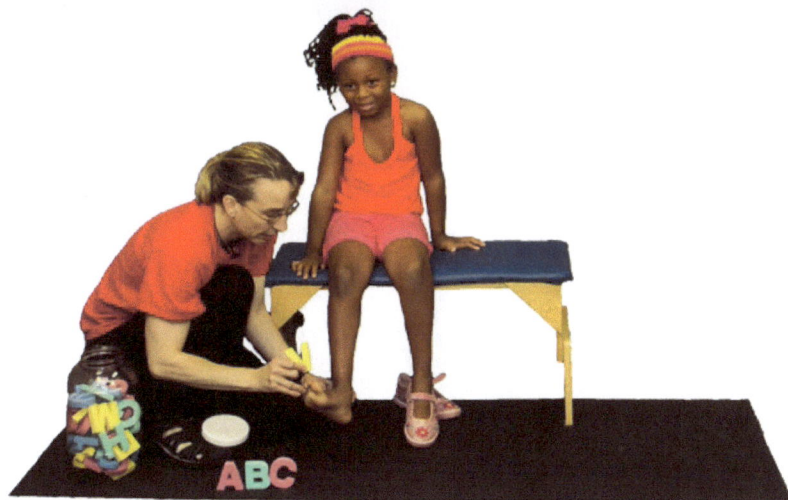

3. SEATED EVERSION, MANUALLY RESISTED

I use the same position as described in the inversion section. I start the child in extreme inversion and cue them to bring their foot into eversion. If a child can get any eversion, it is usually from the extreme inverted position back toward midline. Remember to check a child's passive range first to determine a reasonable end target. Just like with inversion, I perform this activity concentrically and eccentrically.

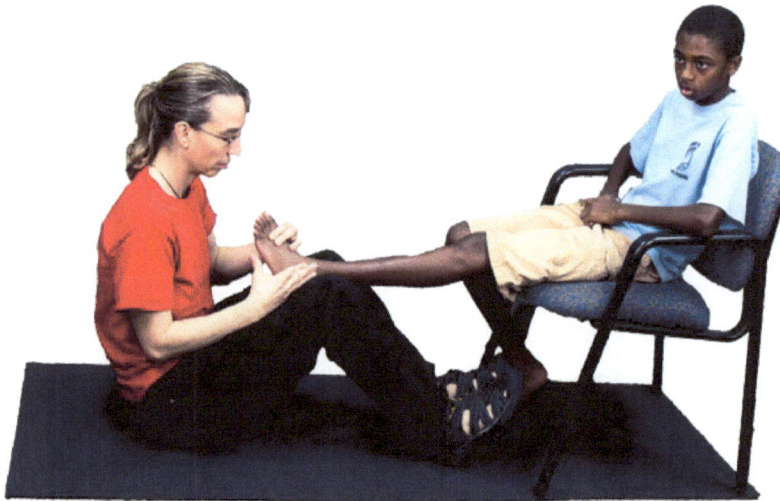

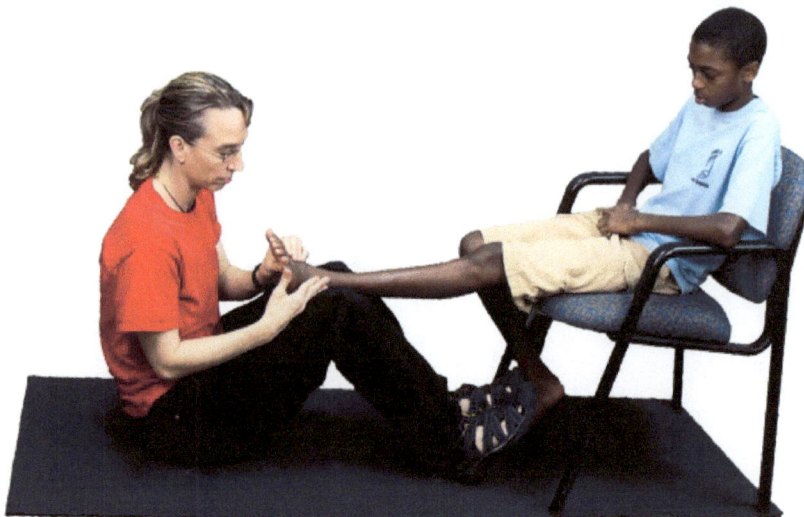

4. EVERSION ELASTIC BAND RESISTANCE

Like the inversion version of this exercise, elastic bands are a good option for graded resistance with a home program. I prefer manual resistance in the clinic. Kids often like the progressively resistant bands for the home program. Sometimes giving clients an object to take home helps make the home program more likely.

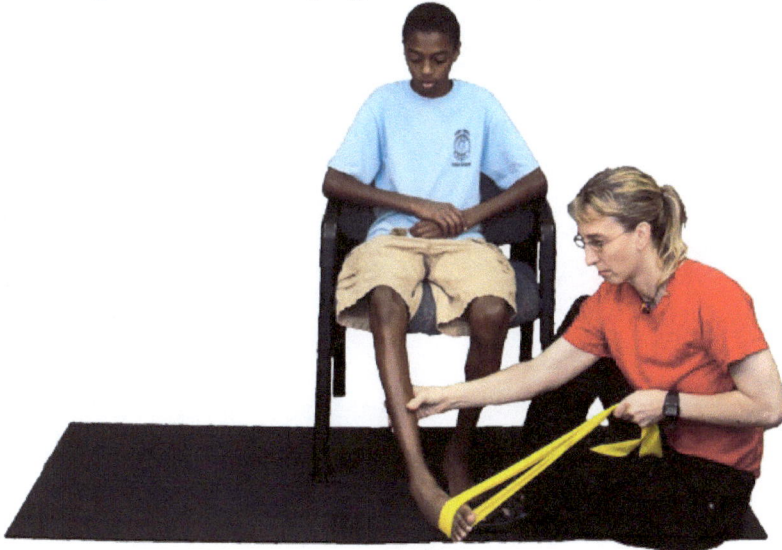

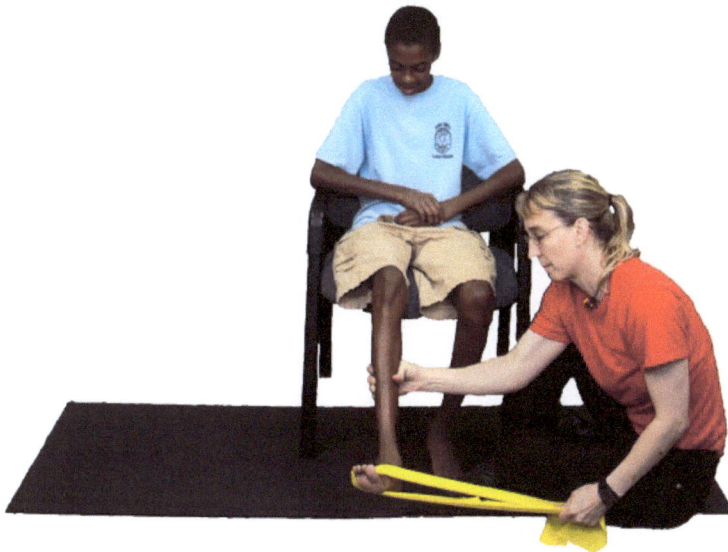

5. SEATED HEEL DOWN EVERSION

This exercise is just the opposite of the one presented in the inversion section. This is where toys with pieces are your friends. Even small children have suffered through this tedious exercise to complete a puzzle or put a car down a ramp. Note how I stabilize the heel to prevent cheating.

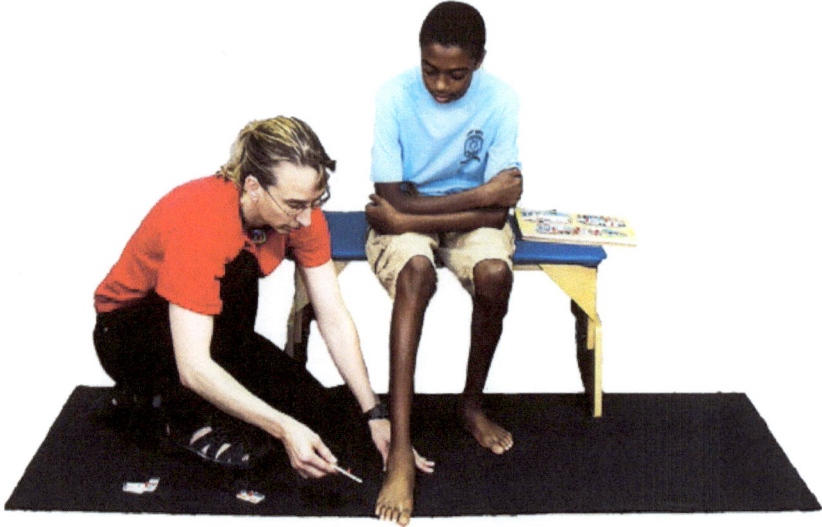

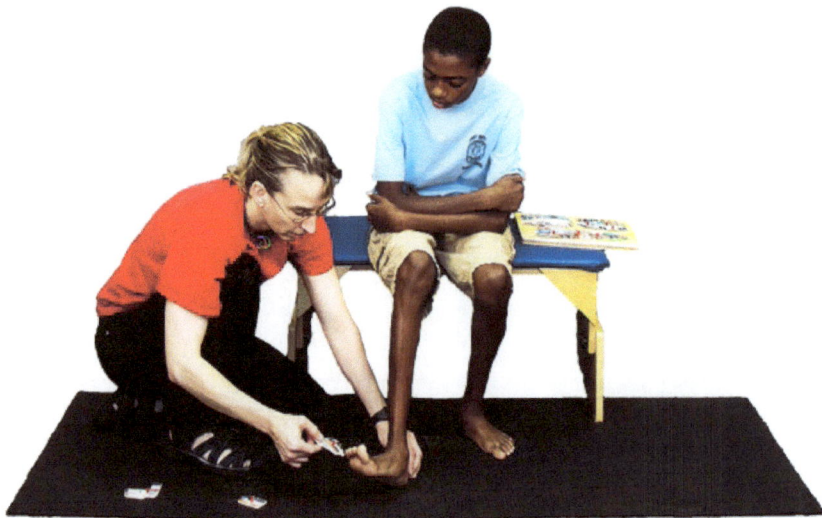

6. SIDEWAYS WIBBLE WOBBLE

This exercise is the same as in the inversion section. If you are trying to get eversion on a particular foot, go the opposite direction as you move across the floor.

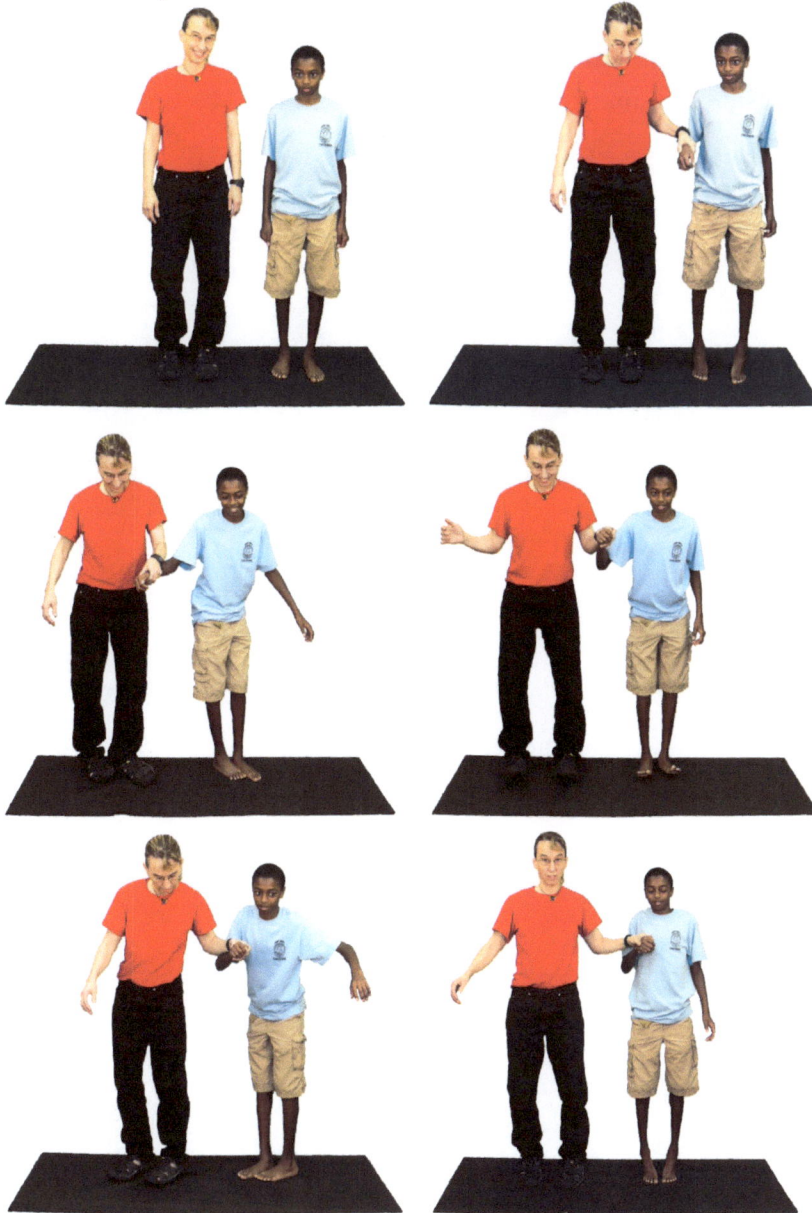

7. STANDING ON A SIDE SLANT

This can be a very challenging exercise. Sometimes I have to start with two hands held, then progress to one hand held, and then to independently. The foot on the downside is working the hardest. It is strongly inverting, but typically the top leg is everting as well. Decrease the slope and the challenge by putting a book under the wedge on the lower side. Document the time the child stands and the angle of the wedge.

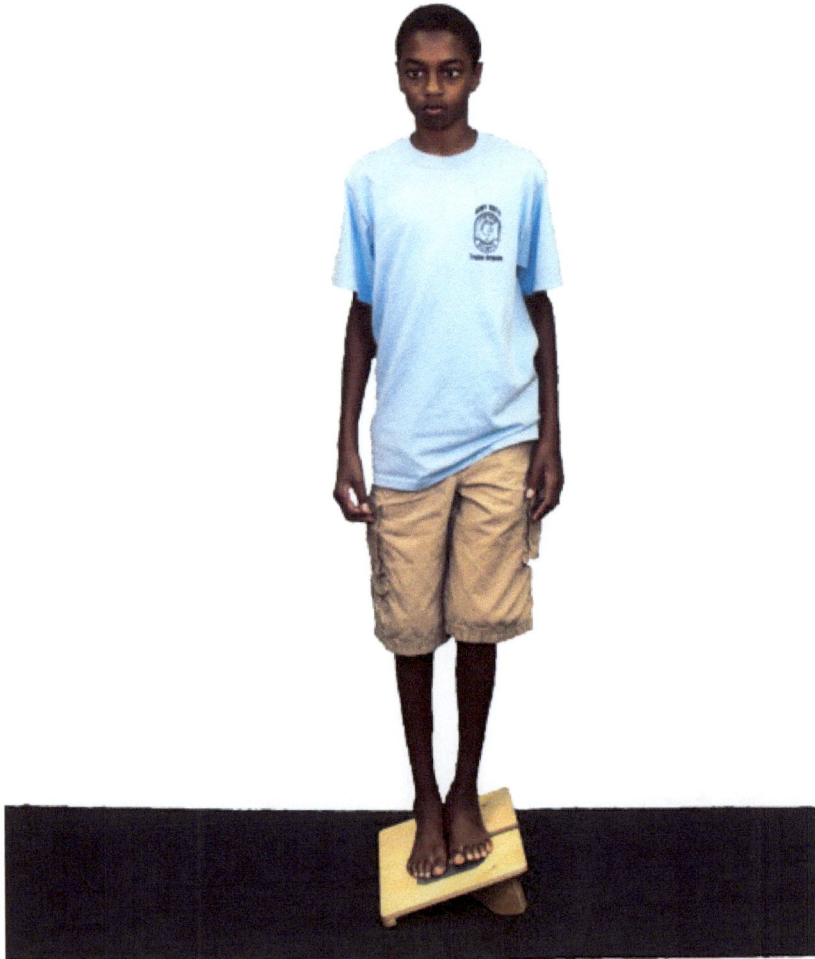

8. ONE LEG SIDE SLANT STAND

Get ready for twice the work when you stand on one leg on the incline. For eversion, the child must stand on the foot closer to the wedge's top as he stands sideways. Again, add appropriate assistance for success. I document similar to the previous exercise.

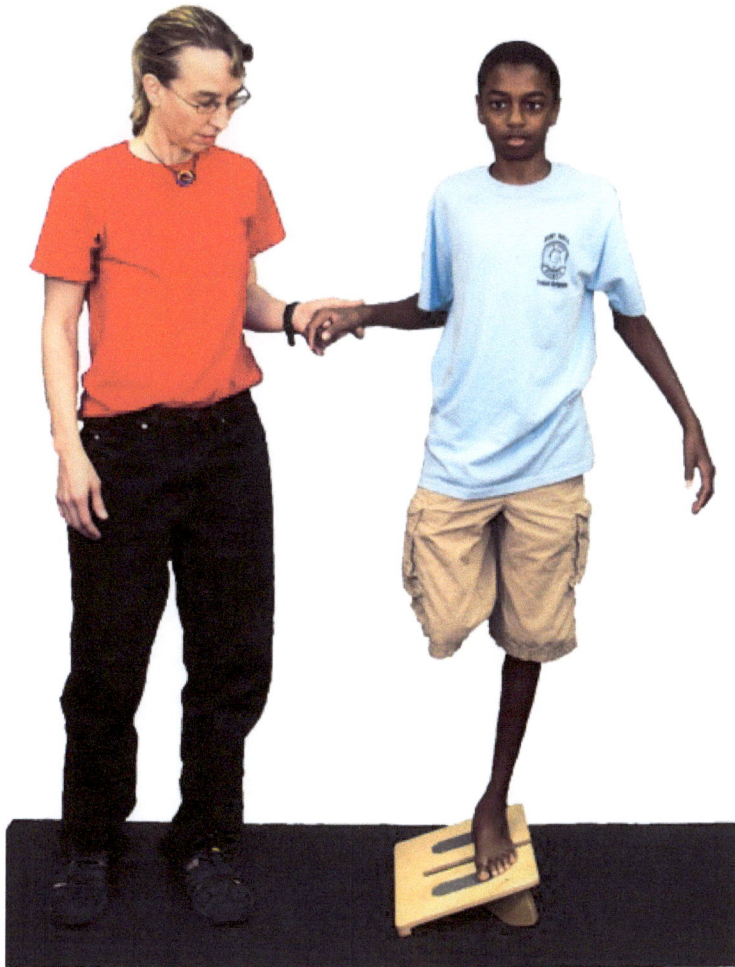

9. STANDING BOLSTER ROLL

This exercise is similar to the one in the inversion chapter. This movement takes a cooperative motivated child to prevent cheating significantly with hip rotation.

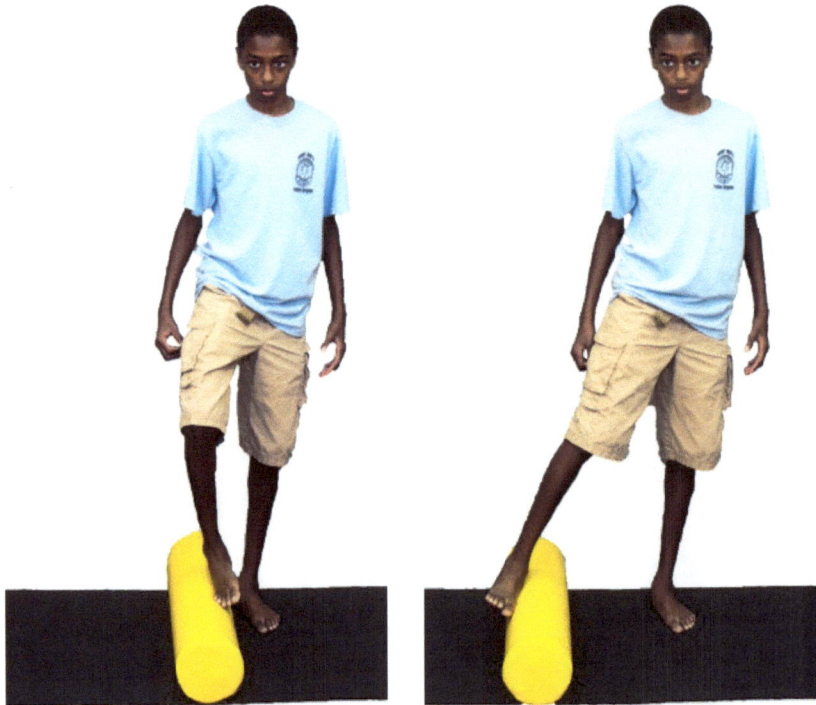

10. STANDING EVERSION KICK

This exercise requires some standing balance unless, of course, you hold a hand or two. The right size bench is essential. If the bench is too small, it is easy to abduct the leg to knock down the target. If it is too large, I end up getting a lot of knee and hip flexion that were not necessarily my goal. The client simply kicks to the side emphasizing foot eversion. Cheating is easy with this exercise, resulting in only hip internal rotation. So this exercise requires a very cooperative client who can concentrate on the proper eversion movement.

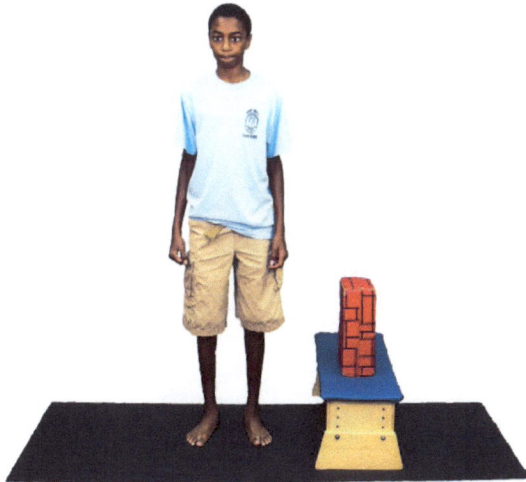

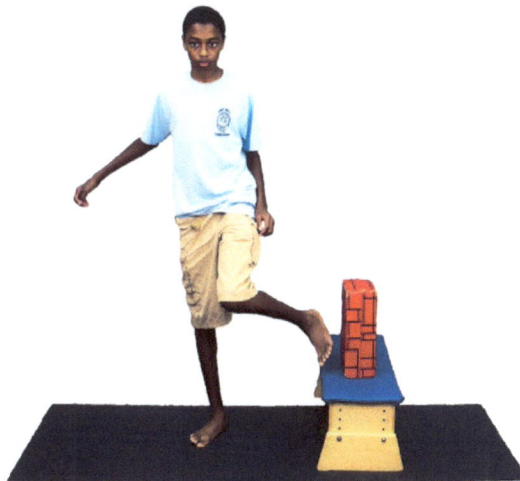

11. STANDING EVERSION ROLLING BALL UP

The proper support and the correct size bench are critical. I like this 16 inch (40 cm) bench, so I can sit on it too. I think my 10-inch (25 cm) bench would work as well, but the 4-inch (10 cm) bench would be too small. A ball with a little traction or texture on it, like a bumpy Gerdy ball, would be easier to control. Again cooperation to prevent an easy cheat with hip rotation is essential.

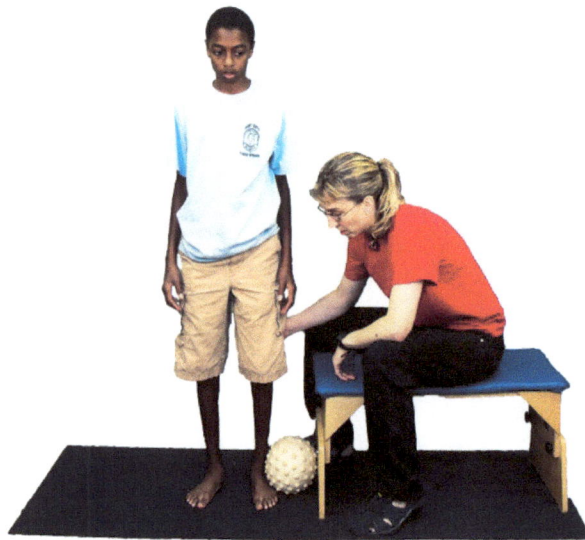

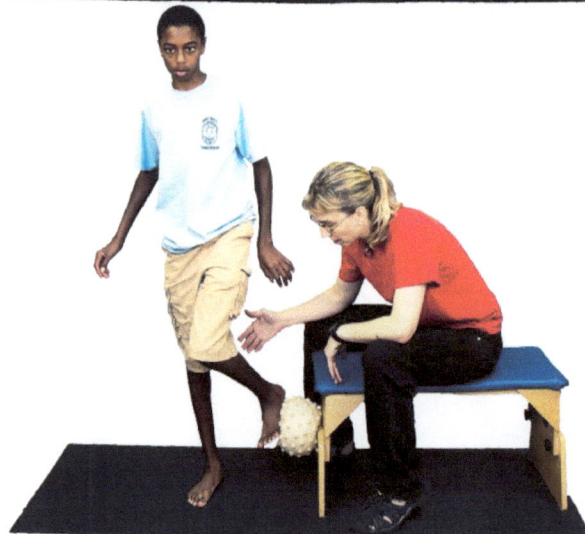

12. STANDING BILATERAL EVERSION

Standing eversion is fairly tricky. When I try it, I always get an overflow of movement at the knee and hip. For picture purposes and ease of clearing the foot's lateral aspect, I had my model place his feet wider. I love using my goniometer to slide under the outside of the foot to confirm the foot's clearance from the floor. For some clients, this activity is more manageable sitting than standing.

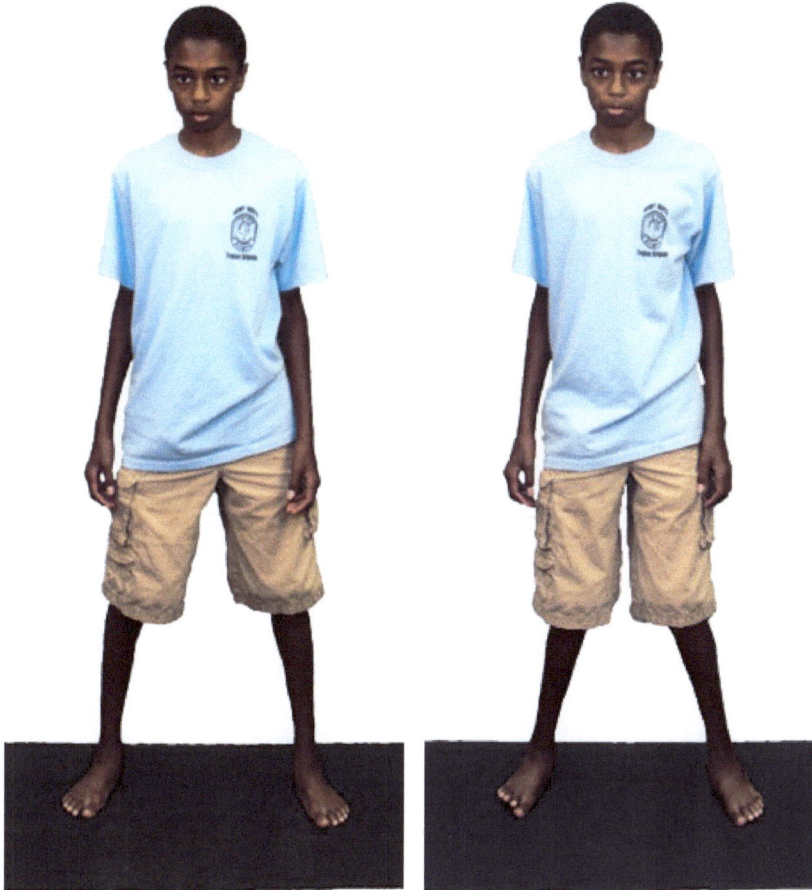

13. SIDE TO SIDE ROCKER BOARD STANDING

I usually start with a client holding on to a support with rocker board work. I progress to no upper body support. I begin with me rocking the board and progress to the client rocking the board independently. To get the repetitions and weight shift I want, I have the client lean to the side to get a strategically placed toy and put it on the other side of the rocker board. I emphasize the child going to end range tilt by putting a keyboard under the rocker board at end range to give an audio cue to indicate that he has gone far enough. I'll do one side for ten repetitions and then place the keyboard on the other side.

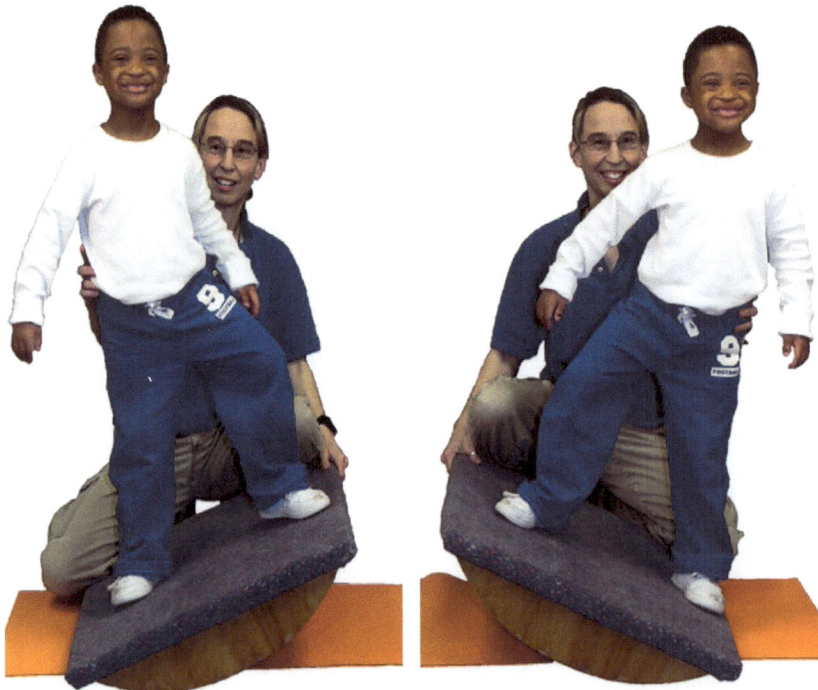

14. SIDE TO SIDE ROCK ON A BALANCE DISC

My directions are similar to those in the inversion section. This
activity tends to get more inversion than eversion activation, but don't
count it out. Remember, it is the higher placed foot that gets more
eversion. The lower foot gets more inversion.

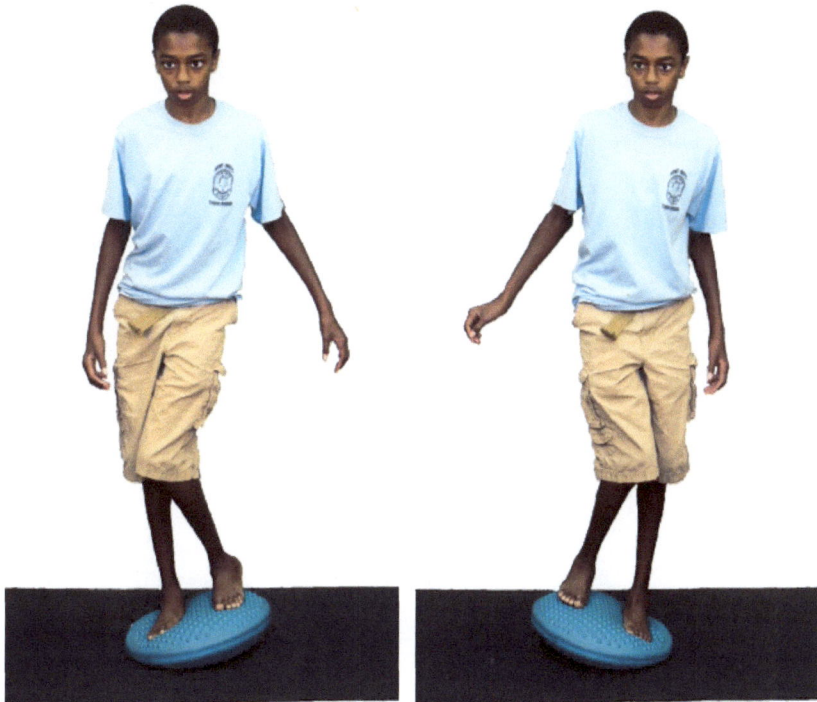

15. SIDE TO SIDE POGO BALL ROCK

Pogo balls allow more extreme rocks in each direction enabling potentially more powerful side to side ankle work. Just balancing on the pogo ball takes strong co-contraction around the ankle joint. Intentional side to side rocking requires power and strength.

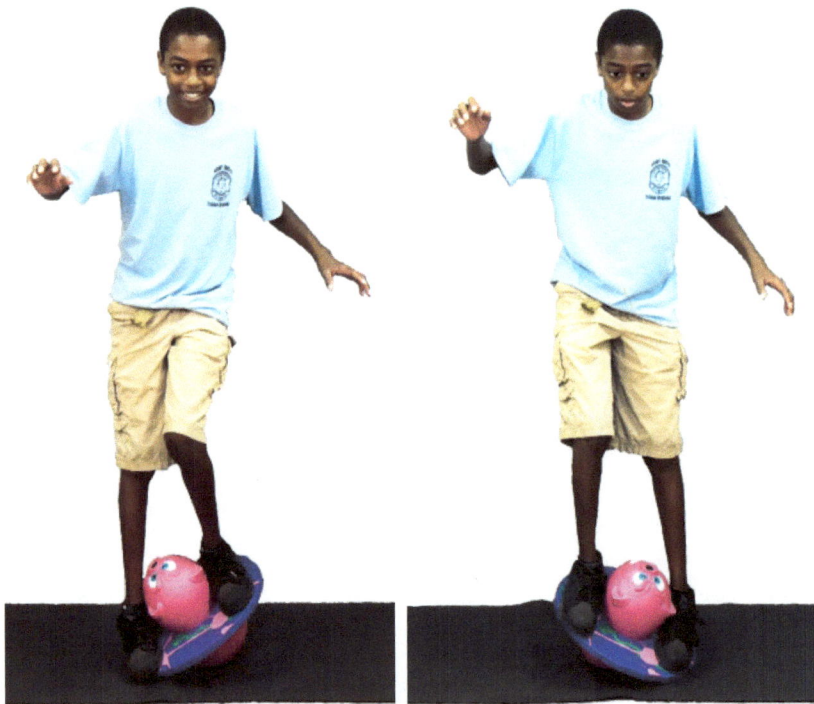

16. IN-LINE STRIDE STANDING

With a narrow base of support, inverters and everters play a larger
role in balance. Remember to keep the feet straight in line for more
isolated inversion and eversion. Tossing a ball or hitting a balloon back
and forth makes this activity more dynamic and encourages muscle
contractions.

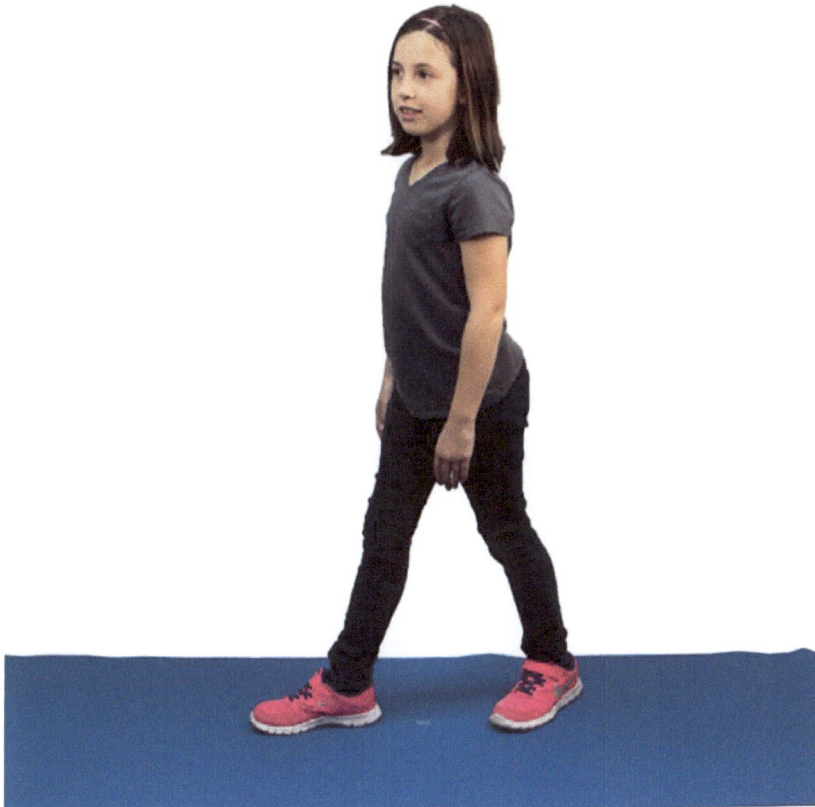

17. SIDE LEAN FROM IN-LINE STRIDE

This exercise works many muscle groups. Included in these are ankle everters, especially on the return to upright. To make this easier, go down to a bench instead of the floor. Try to keep the feet straight for more isolated inversion/eversion.

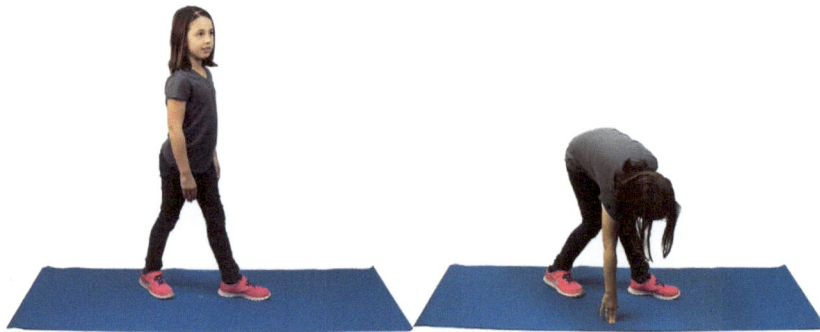

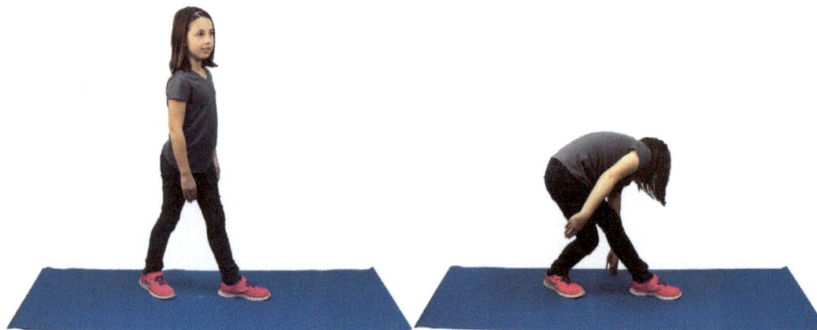

18. STANDING ON ONE FOOT

Standing on one foot is good for developing inversion/eversion strength, but standing on one foot while performing a dynamic activity is even better.

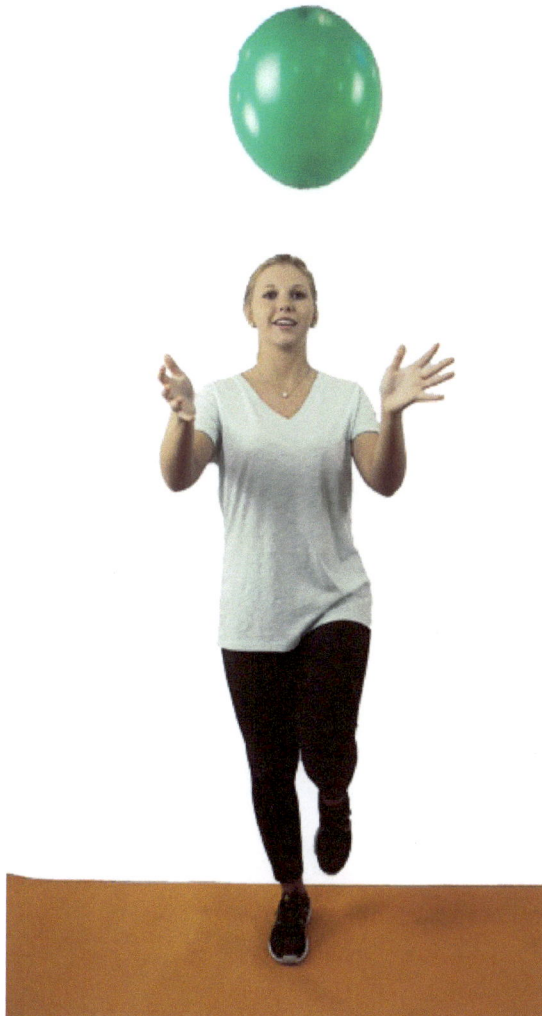

19. SINGLE LEG STANCE PENDULUM SWINGS

To ensure powerful muscle contractions of inversion and eversion, pendulum swings of the free leg in the sagittal plane do quite nicely. Quicker movements to a metronome beat would challenge most people. Add an ankle weight on the moving leg to the mix to create a challenging variation.

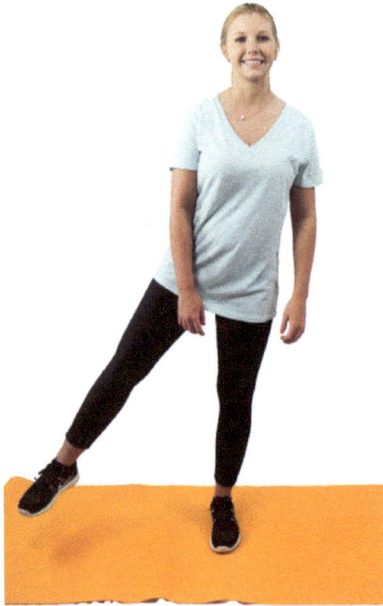

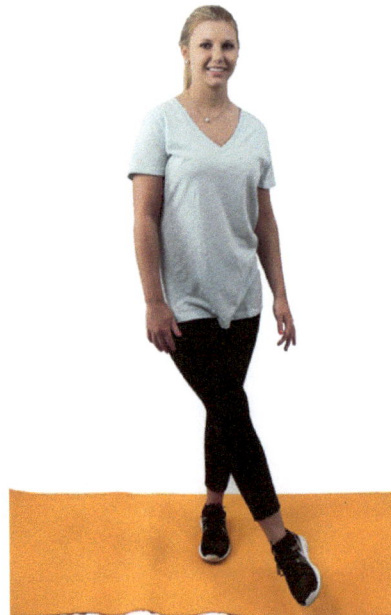

PEDIATRIC PHYSICAL THERAPY STRENGTHENING EXERCISES FOR THE ANKLES

OTHER BOOKS BY THE AUTHOR

A is for Autism

D is for Down Syndrome

C is for Cerebral Palsy

A is for Attention Deficit Hyperactivity Disorder

Pediatric Physical Therapy Strengthening Exercises for the Hips

Pediatric Physical Therapy Strengthening Exercises for the Knees

ABOUT THE AUTHOR

AMY STURKEY IS AN OUTPATIENT pediatric physical therapist at Child and Family Development in Charlotte, NC. Amy met a family with an adorable boy with cerebral palsy on a safari in Kenya. As she tried to help them, she realized that little information was available to help train pediatric therapists and to educate children and families about common childhood conditions and treatment options. Determined to share her 30+ years of clinical experience, she co-founded Gotcha Apps to produce educational products for pediatric therapists and their clients. She created a Facebook page (Pediatric Physical Therapy Exercises), a web-site, and a YouTube channel (Pediatric Physical Therapy Exercises). Through these platforms, she releases weekly videos to instruct therapists and families of children with developmental challenges. Amy won Outstanding Physical Therapist for North Carolina for 2016. Her books are available on Amazon, Kindle, Audible, and in the Apple Library.

www.PediatricPTexercises.com

www.ingramcontent.com/pod-product-compliance
Lightning Source LLC
Chambersburg PA
CBHW060807270326
41927CB00003B/77